Your

PROSTATE

Its Functions and Malfunctions
As Well As All Known
Methods of

TREATMENT and PREVENTION

by the same author

GROWING FLOWERS
GARDEN GLIMPSES
ROMANCE IN THE GARDEN
HUNZA: ADVENTURES IN A LAND OF PARADISE
THE ART OF GROWING DWARF POTTED TREES
LET'S MAKE OUR OWN WINES AND BEERS
MILK -- FRIEND OR FIEND?
ENZYMES -- THE SPARK OF LIFE
HYDROGENATION -- AMERICA'S DEADLIEST KILLER
ASPIRIN -- MONSTER IN DISGUISE
EAT RIGHT AND BE HEALTHY
PROVEN HERBAL REMEDIES
SALT AND YOUR HEALTH
BANISH BACKACHE
"NO-COOK" BOOK
GUIDEPOSTS TO HEALTH AND VIGOROUS LONG LIFE
SPROUTS -- ELIXIR OF LIFE

YOUR
PROSTATE

Its functions and malfunctions as well as all known methods of

TREATMENT
AND
PREVENTION

TWO VOLUMES IN ONE

-- o --

PUBLISHED IN CANADA

1st Printing; Aug. 1967
2nd Printing; Nov. 1967
3rd Printing; Jan. 1968
4th Printing; Dec. 1968
5th Printing; Aug. 1969
6th Printing; Jan. 1970
7th Printing; Feb. 1971
8th Printing, Sept. 1971

PROVOKER PRESS
St. Catharines, Ontario

TABLE OF CONTENTS

Book One

Chapter		Page
	Introduction	xv
1.	Description and Functions of the Prostate	1
2.	Disorders and Malfunctions of the Prostate	17
3.	Symptoms	27
4.	Is Prostate Trouble a Disease of Old Age?	35
5.	What is Retention?	45
6.	Causes of Prostate Disorders	55
7.	Food Additives and the Prostate	93
8.	Meat Eating and Its Effects Upon the Prostate	103
9.	Sex and Your Prostate	111
10.	Fear -- Its Role in Prostate Disorders	141
11.	Catheters and Catheterization	149
12.	Preventive Measures	157

13. Recurrence 161

14. Hold Everything! It May Not Be Your Prostate! 167

15. Abstinence and Homosexuality 177

16. Personal History 183

17. The Prostate and Senility 193

18. Are Wives to Blame? 203

19. Coitus Prolongatus 207

20. Coitus Interruptus 211

21. Coitus Reservatus 219

22. The Danger of Forcing the Orgasm 229

23. The Last Post 233

24. Summary 239

Book Two

Introduction 255

1. Water Treatment 259

2. Herbal Methods 261

3. Osteopathic Methods 265

4. Surgical Methods 273

5. Modern Medical Methods 285

6. Older Medical Methods 299

7. Treating Prostatic Hypertrophy with Vitamin F 315

8. Homeopathic Methods 325

9. The Hygienic System for Prostate Disorder 331

10. Wheat Grass Method of Treatment 337

11. Yogi Therapy for an Enlarged Prostate 339

12. Naturopathic Methods 343

13. Chiropractic Treatment 349

14. Ayurvedic Treatment (From India) 361

15. The Author's Counsel 363

Glossary 379

Bibliography 383

LIST OF ILLUSTRATIONS

Facing Page

The Anatomy of the Urethra .... (xiii)

Normal Prostate and Related Organs 51

Enlarged Prostate and Related Organs ... 51

Median Section of the Male Pelvis 62

Distended Bladder and Other Organs 110

Seminal Vesicles 111

Catheters in Place 148

Normal Kidneys 156

Affected Kidneys 157

Pelvic Structures 166

Supra-pubic Prostatectomy 272

Transurethral Prostatectomy 276

Retro-pubic Prostatectomy 280

Perineal Prostatectomy 282

He who with swift, unerring hand,
Has oft removed a prostate gland,
Has reaped the harvest he has sown --
He's having trouble with his own.

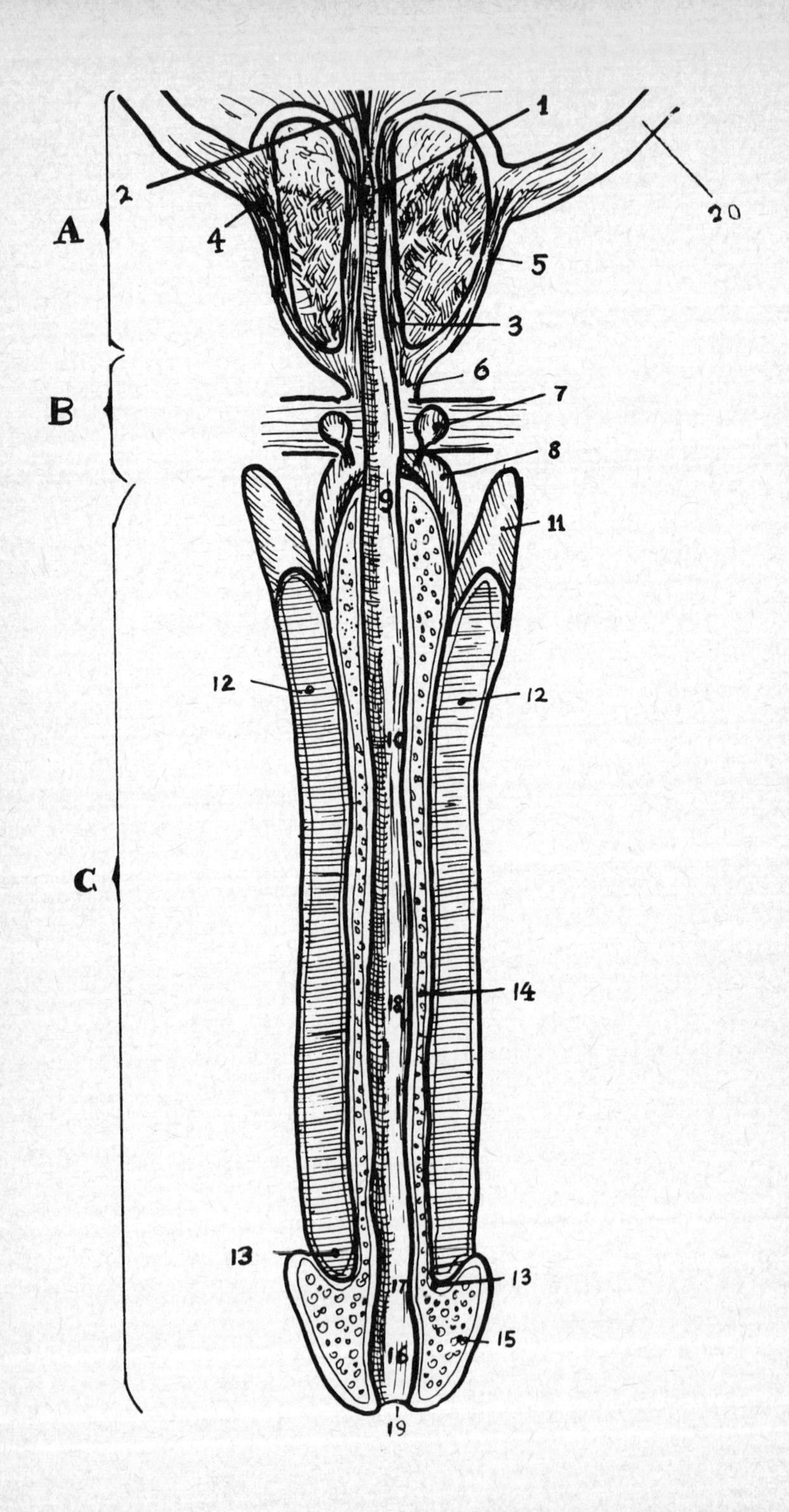

A
B
C
1
2
3
4
5
6
7
8
9
10
11
12
12
13
13
14
15
16
17
18
19
20

THE ANATOMY OF THE URETHRA

The urethra opened along its upper surface, and spread out in order to show the details of its interior and lateral surfaces.

A, Prostatic portion; B, membranous portion; C, spongy portion.

1, Verumontanum, with the orifices of the ejaculatory ducts; 2, frenum of the verumontanum; 3, prostate, with the prostatic glandules; 4, section through the unstriped sphincter; 5, section through the striped sphincter; 6, wall of the membranous portion; 7, Cowper's glands, with, 7, the orifices of their ducts; 8, bulb; 9, longitudinal folds of the bulbous and membranous portions of the urethra; 10, posterior wall of the spongy urethra; 11, roots of the corpora cavernosa; 12, septum between the corpora cavernosa, along which the urethra has been opened; 12', orifice, or lacuna, through which the meshes of the two corpora cavernosa intercommunicate; 13, termination of the corpus cavernosum in an excavation in the glans; 13', fibrous septum separating corpus cavernosum from glans; 14, section through the anterior part of the corpus cavernosum; 15, glans; 16, fossa navicularis, with 17, the two halves of Guerin's valve; 18, lacunae of Morgagni; 19, meatus; 20, bladder wall.

INTRODUCTION

The simple fact that you are reading this book indicates that you may already be suffering from a prostate disorder or that you have seen or felt signs that indicate all is not well with your genitals and bladder. I cannot visualize any individual seeking knowledge on the prostate unless it has already given him cause for concern. So there is no doubt about it, this book is meant for you.

While it is generally conceded that the number one killer in the Western world is heart disease, followed by cancer, this does not alter the fact that more males suffer from prostate disorders than from heart trouble and cancer combined. The figures that I have been able to obtain concerning the number of prostatic sufferers are not conclusive. I have sought information from many sources and questioned many medical men in various parts of the country. This I will say ... detailed information on the number of prostate cases is very difficult to obtain.

However, I feel quite secure in stating that at least 70% of all males over 50 have already had some trouble with their prostate gland. At age 60 the incidence of prostate trouble in males would rise to almost 85% and at age 70 and over, the incidence, in my opinion, would run close to or even above 90%.

My investigations would lead me to believe that seldom does a man past 70 years of age fail to have some form of trouble with his prostate gland. There's no doubt about it -- not one man in 10 past 70 is free of prostate trouble.

If, in buying this book, it was your hope to find a quick and easy cure for your prostate disorder, I want to disillusion you right now. There is no such thing as a quick and easy cure for disorders of this gland. However, if you are seeking truth, if you are trying to find out the causes or contributing factors involved in prostate disorders, I believe this work will be of help. If you are seeking guidance, if you desire information concerning problems that face the prostate sufferer, then I believe you have come to the right source.

Now this may sound like wishful thinking but I contend that within the pages of this book I have outlined practically all of the factors involved in causing prostate disorders.

Chapter One

DESCRIPTION AND FUNCTIONS OF THE PROSTATE

I have read and heard many definitions of the prostate gland. One of the best, in my opinion, refers to it as "the male motor," suggesting that it is the motivating force in the human male structure. It is sometimes called the "sexual brain." Here are some other names that could describe this complex and important gland -- the male womb, the male axis, the male generator, the vital male gland.

No one can deny that it is a complex organ combining physical, psychic and sexual aspects. Writers and students keep stressing that it is the most important of the sexual organs but it must not be considered in but one of its many miens ... all of its different functions and aspects must be studied.

It seems that there is some confusion between the word "prostate" and the term "prostate gland." Actually, no one seems to be positively sure of the proper term. One authority states that, strictly speaking, in referring to the muscle and gland parts in combination it is proper to refer to it as the prostate rather than the prostate gland, because once muscle tissue and other facets are involved it is better to leave out the word "gland." It is estimated that only 1/4 to 1/3 of the prostate is made up of glandular tissue. Therefore, the term "gland" is not exactly proper or correct. I understand that even among physicians the terms "prostate" and "prostate gland" are used a bit too loosely.

One eminent authority claims, "There is evidence to suggest the prostate is a ductless gland, though this has not been substantiated. Nevertheless the prostate appears to be closely related to the ductless glands and thus can produce far-reaching effects when prostate troubles occur."

In all the literature that I have studied about the prostate I found it was invariably compared to a chestnut in shape, but nowhere did they specify whether it was a horse chestnut or a sweet chestnut and these nuts have distinctly different shapes. The horse chestnut is oval and spheroid whereas the sweet chestnut is distinctly cone or wedge shaped. Therefore, I suggest that the prostatic gland has the form or shape of a large sweet chestnut.

The prostate is a firm, partly glandular, partly muscular organ, situated in the pelvis, at the base of the bladder, surrounding the urethra, and pierced by the urethra at its origin from the urinary bladder. It is the size of a large sweet chestnut, somewhat conical in shape, measuring approximately one and a half inches wide, three quarters of an inch from front to back, and one and three eighths inches high, and weighing about 25 grams. It contains about thirty to fifty small glands which drain through sixteen to thirty small ducts into the urethra, after passing through the upper posterior portion of the prostate. In these small gland cavities is secreted a mucus fluid manufactured by the prostate and therein is also stored the semen from the testicles. These glands are activated by male hormones. Some authorities suggest that the prostate produces the male sex hormones but this has not been positively established.

The following description of the prostate is the best I could locate and although a bit technical, it does give the best detail ... thus, I am using it. The glossary at the back of the book will explain any of the troublesome words.

"The prostate is a sexual gland, its secretion being mixed with the sperm in the urethra at the time of ejaculation, and functioning to activate and prolong the motility of the spermatozoa. The gland has five lobes (median, two lateral, posterior, and anterior), and a group of gland acini in the midline of the urethral floor between the posterior vesical lip and the verumontanum (the subcervical urethral glands of Albarran). The median lobe is that part dorsal to the urethra and between the converging ejaculatory ducts. The median lobe, the glands of Albarran, and the lateral lobes are particularly prone to undergo benign enlargement and cause obstruction."

The prostate gland fits neatly around the neck or base of the bladder just where the urethra begins. It can best be described by saying it encompasses the proximal urethra which is the urinary canal. The urethra is the membranous tube through which the urine flows. There is a vital relationship between the bladder, the rectum and the prostate. The apex of the prostate lies about one and a half inches away from the anus.

The two lateral lobes and the middle lobe of the prostate are made of glandular as well as muscular tissue. The base of the prostatic urethra and its strong muscular tissue form a wall of great firmness and strength through which flow the many prostatic ducts. The tubes of these ducts carry the fluid prostatic secretions for distribution with seminal secretions as required during sexual relations and ultimate ejaculation.

Through the central lobe of the prostate pass the two ejaculatory ducts and these empty into the urethra where at the appropriate time the prostatic fluid is mixed with the secretions from the seminal vesicles. The seminal fluid, mixed with other secretions, is propelled by means of the contracting fibrous prostate muscles through the urethra and into the prepared or occupied orifice.

The purpose of the ejaculation and the ejaculatory ducts is (1) to buckshot the semen so that it will be more likely to penetrate the uterus, (2) to prevent the semen, which coagulates rather quickly, from remaining in the urethra or the meatus, (3) to render the male somewhat immobile so that he will not withdraw and defeat nature's purpose, and (4) to prevent and counter other actions on the part of the male so that he will better perform nature's function.

The urinary system is composed of the following organs: kidneys, ureters, bladder and urethra. I cannot definitely establish whether the prostate gland is considered a part of the urinary system but it is certainly involved in the actions and functions of that system.

The bladder holds one-half to one pint (that is, 8 to 16 ounces) and under certain circumstances will hold up to one quart of fluid. The urethra generally averages approximately 6 1/2 inches in length, of which the first 1 1/4 inches at the neck of the bladder passes through a deep furrow in the prostate gland. This is sometimes referred to as the prostatic urethra.

I have heard the prostate referred to as the controlling valve of the urinary bladder. While the urinary bladder is being filled in the general course of events within the body, the prostate, in conjunction with the sphincter muscles, keeps the valve shut tightly. When the bladder is ready for emptying and the body calls upon it to empty, the sphincter-prostate team opens the valve and the flow begins.

The prostate is the focal point of the sexual organs. Make no mistake about it, all of the organs that surround the prostate are vitally important and each plays its part and makes its contribution to the welfare of the body as a whole. But not one of them is as vital or as important as the prostate itself. It is upon the prostate that the male depends not only for sexual gratification but for desire, drive and stamina.

At this point I will try to explain in the simples possible language the functions and inter-relationships of the various sex glands and organs so that you might better understand their contribution towards the well-being of the male body.

The testicles manufacture the spermatozoa and supposedly form an internal secretion or hormone which is considered to be partially responsible for sex desire as well as promoting the development of the secondary sexual characteristics ... muscular strength, hair on the face, a deep voice and other typically masculine features.

The actual production of the spermatozoa supposedly takes place in the tiny tubules of the testicles, and there are a goodly number of these tubules -- at the least, well over 1,000. This process is known as spermatogenesis. A healthy, fully mature spermatozoon, when viewed under a microscope, can be seen to have a head, neck and tail ... in general appearance and form, it resembles a polliwog. However, at this stage it is rather inactive.

When the spermatozoa have reached full development they circulate through the tubules into a collecting duct which finally carries them into two receptacles, known as the seminal vesicles, that are located on either side of the prostate. These seminal vesicles act as a storehouse for the accumulation of the completely formed spermatozoa. In the actual act of an orgasm these reservoirs force the spermatozoa through a tiny canal into the urethra where they are flooded in prostatic secretion.

Evidently the secretion of the prostate acts as a spark, for as soon as the spermatozoa are covered with the prostatic solution they spring to life and feverish activity. They are often described as acting like tadpoles in a puddle -- but not until they come in contact with the prostatic secretion. This mixture is then referred to as the semen or the seminal fluid.

It is claimed that up to 200,000,000 spermatozoa are ejaculated when an orgasm is reached. When you realize that but one spermatozoon is required to effect fertilization, you will see that nature does not gamble or leave anything to chance.

Now at this point I'd like to alert my readers so that they will not confuse the functions of the prostate gland with those of the testicles or gonads, as they are properly known. The gonads, in addition to manufacturing the spermatozoa, produce a secretion which is constantly fed into the blood stream and carried by the blood to every part of the body.

There is no doubt that the prostate and the gonads are linked in some manner. This co-existence is irrefutable. Both produce vital fluids, both contribute to man's masculinity and fecundity ... but precisely how they are controlled and operated has yet to be discovered. However, we do know that by working in harmony they combine to produce the seminal fluid and at the opportune moment to deposit it where it belongs when a couple indulge in normal sexual relationship.

From the age of puberty until the time of the male climacteric, the process of spermatogenesis continues unceasingly, while the male is in good health. So to sum it up in simple language, we could say that a man is considered virile or fertile from approximately 15 years of age right up until 50 or 60 or even 70, depending upon the health of the individual. But it is not unusual to find men past 80 who still produce active spermatozoa in their bodies.

It is believed, but without positive proof, that the prostate gland also produces and excretes an internal secretion that acts in conjunction with the interstitial secretion of the gonads in maintaining masculine virility. Some writers like to compare prostate disorders with the menopause in women ... after the age of 50 the hypertrophy of the gland is a normal development and when this condition arises, this fluid and its resulting manifestations cease to function -- thus reducing or eliminating sexual desire as is supposed to be the case when women have their menopause. This is subsequently believed to be a condition arising due to the advance of age.

The greater the desire for sex, the more intense the psychic emotion, the more profuse will be this secretion. Thus, it is characteristic that this secretion flows more profusely in the early years of virile life and diminishes in amount with the encroachment of old age. Some authorities attribute this function to the prostate gland, but I do not agree.

Whether or not the prostate has any connection with or contributes anything towards the function of the Cowper's glands, no one seems to know. However it does manufacture a secretion ... but precisely what this secretion does is not fully understood. It is believed that it coats the genital and urinary canal with a lubricating agent. Thus, when the semen is ejaculated, its passage is made rapid and unimpeded. Furthermore, this essential secretion is mucilaginous in nature and continually spreads and covers the sensitive lining of the prostate canal and thus protects its tender nerves, cells and duct openings against irritation by the flow of urine.

Every virile, normal male has at one time or another, when sexually aroused, felt an oily excretion that seeped from the urethra. In my youth, when this happened to me for the first few times, I thought it was actually a premature ejaculation. But of course I soon learned that it was nature's way of preparing the organ for sexual intercourse. It is normal and proper that when a male is sexually aroused this secretion should appear. It is a well-known fact that this mucilaginous, slippery, oily substance is prepared by nature to keep the organ well oiled to permit easy entrance into the vaginal canal of the female. Some authorities say that this oil should appear when intensely or violently sexually aroused but it is my contention that even normal desire should produce this lubricant. However, it is not established whether this secretion is produced by the prostate or by the Cowper's glands or by a combination of both.

It is believed by many authorities that this fluid fulfills the same function as does the secretion of the Bartholin glands in the female which also pour out a pre-coital fluid which is intended to lubricate the vagina in preparation for the act of coitus.

One authority claims that the prostate gland is the soul of sexual life and thus, any problem which affects this gland is regarded with deep concern, if not dismay.

It is related that in the process of intercourse the blood pressure within the prostatic blood vessels is greatly increased and this, in turn, causes a noticeable swelling in the prostate. During this procedure an adequate supply of prostatic fluid is generated. The greater the pressure brought about by the prostate the more desirable and essential it becomes for the male to complete the sexual act by ejaculation and this, I contend, is one of the foremost purposes of the prostate. Then, and then only, is its function logically and biologically fulfilled.

What the male knows as the ejaculation process is actually created by the forceful contraction of the prostate. The prostate functions like a piston and actually hurls the semen from the opening of the penis. In this

way it is widely scattered throughout the vagina with the intent of penetrating the uterus of the female.

A major part of the prostate structure is made up of involuntary muscle fibre and thus no conscious control is held over it. However, the prostate as an entity is in partial control and sometimes when grossly enlarged or inflamed, is in complete control of the bladder. Then we have retention of the urine. The muscles function automatically and over this we have a form of control -- at least some men learn to control it -- for example, when we temporarily withhold an orgasm.

It is by means of the prostate that some men acquire the ability to gain control over the duration of the sexual act. A healthy prostate will permit great flexibility concerning the duration of the sex act. A weak or poorly functioning prostate will give rise to premature ejaculation, resulting in totally unsatisfactory sexual relations for both partners. This is referred to as coitus praecox.

It is a strange phenomenon -- to me at least -- that such vital organs as the gonads are left exposed so openly in all animals, whereas the prostate is located within the body where it is well protected. Evidently nature felt that the prostate and its functions were more vital than the gonads. Please remember that this is just a conjecture.

I have known innumerable boys and men who, through the years, suffered varying injuries to their testicles and I doubt if a male can grow from infancy to old age without having some form of injury, no matter how slight, to his testicles. I took part in various athletic sports when I was a lad -- baseball, basketball, skating, football, running, jumping -- and somewhere along in these activities I ran into kicks, punches and other incidents that gave me pain or concern with my testicles. So again I say that nature certainly did not shield these glands very carefully. I have often wondered why.

The only cxplanation that came my way through my diligent searching was that the testicles must be kept at a lower temperature than the rest of the body in order for them to function properly. Thus, being suspended from the body, the 98.6 degree normal body temperature does not apply to the gonads.

The fluid that the prostate gland secretes has a most profound influence upon the function and activity of the entire male body. It is believed that the prostate does have a close relationship to other vital organs of the body, such as the pituitaries, the thyroid and the adrenals.

The prostate also greatly affects the individual's personality. Some people maintain that a man who is without a prostate is but a shell of a man -- timorous, lacking in zest and purpose of life. Some even go so far as to say that he is continually in ill humor, peevish and an all-round weakling. However, there is no proof that this holds true. Personally I know many men who have never had the slightest trouble with their prostate yet they are just as described.

Somewhere along in my studies it was pointed out that those men who had a weak prostate, and thus also a low incidence of sex, were pessimists while those who had a strong prostate and a high incidence of sex were optimists. Please do not apply this as a general rule of thumb, but it is well worth some consideration and investigation.

When the prostate gland is not functioning as it should, both the urinary and the sexual performances are disturbed. Therefore, it must be reflected in the individual's behaviour, his outlook, his thoughts, his temperament and his entire way of life. A strong prostate in perfect condition gives a man a feeling of superiority. When the gland is sick or in trouble, then he has a feeling of inferiority. I contend that the prostate affects the whole wide spectrum of a man's horizon.

It is generally accepted and conceded that sexual virility is synonymous with bodily power. I don't know just how true this statement is but certainly if one is not in good health, it is difficult or next to impossible to perform the sex act satisfactorily ... that is, for any extended period. Broadly speaking, physical strength is indicative of sexual vigor ... but this does not necessarily mean that the biggest men are the most virile men!

Of all the various powers that man possesses none is more important psychologically than his sexual power or as it is also called, his virility. It has been claimed, yet disputed, that the more potent a man is sexually the greater is the drive within him and the greater his worldly achievements. There is no doubt about it, there is some connection, some vital link between a man's accomplishments and his virility.

Here I am going to enumerate the known functions of the prostate. While the prostate may not in itself control or create all of these activities, it does take either the leading or an important part in them...

1. Assisting in creating or maintaining an erection of the penis.
2. Instrumental in the performance of the ejaculation.
3. Activating the seminal fluid.
4. Controlling the flow of urine in conjunction with the sphincter muscles of the bladder.
5. Controlling the duration of the sexual act.
6. Controlling the frequency of the sexual act.
7. Providing or assisting to provide the lubricating fluid for the sexual act.
8. Contributing to the control of the emotions.
9. Motivating force in all male activities.

Nature evidently anticipated the tremendous burden that would be placed upon the prostate for she endowed this gland and its contiguous tissue with a large mass of

nerve fibre as well as a copious supply of blood. Evidently the concentration of blood, nerve fibre and nerve supply makes the prostate susceptible to congestion and varied glandular malfunctions.

To sum up, let us examine the heavy load that the prostate must bear. It must open and shut the valves many times during the day for the passage of the urine. It must prepare for and be ready at short notice for the seminal flow. It must at regular or frequent intervals bring about the desire for sexual relations. It must control and help perform these relations. It must have at all times a supply of preparatory and other secretions. It must at a given instant bring pressure to bear and function like a piston to expel the seminal fluid from the meatus.

So, all in all, you can understand that the prostate does have a great deal of work to perform.

Chapter Two

DISORDERS AND MALFUNCTIONS OF THE PROSTATE

It is one of the peculiar things about human nature that when a man has an upset stomach or a bit of dust in his eye or an ache in his shoulder or head or back, he will quickly consult his healer . . . but when the most vital organ in his body begins to cause trouble, he hides his discomfort and keeps it to himself. Of course, the reason is not too hard to understand. We are somewhat embarrassed or ashamed to admit that we are having trouble with our genital organs and we don't like doctors, nurses or technicians fooling about with them. Therefore, a man tends to avoid broadcasting his distress or even confiding in or consulting anyone concerning this often serious personal ailment.

Often men suffer with prostatic enlargement in silence until they can endure it no longer and by then, in many cases, the condition has become so far advanced that it is hopeless for anything else but drastic surgery. My warning to all of those who begin to have difficulty or problems that in any way affect the prostate is to seek counsel promptly. It need not necessarily be from a physician. There are many other qualified practitioners in the various fields of healing who could be consulted. There are also many good books on health that cover the subject quite thoroughly. The big, the important thing is to get competent advice and guidance as quickly as possible.

I have tried to get facts and figures concerning the number of men afflicted with prostate trouble in its various forms but I found that these statistics are practically impossible to obtain.

I sought to establish percentage figures but they varied so greatly from informant to informant that it left scant basis for anything of a concrete nature.

The lowest percentage that was quoted from any source was that 40% of all males 50 years old and over had some form of prostate trouble. The highest percentage was 85% when referring to males 50 years of age and over. My own opinion, from all the information I have received, is that probably 70% of all males over 50 is closer to the correct figure. This would suggest that at least seven out of every ten men over 50 years of age in Canada and the United States are suffering from various forms or degrees of prostate trouble.

One authority claims that the prostate is the most troublesome of all the male organs. The suggested figure that 70% or more of all males over 50 years of age are suffering from some malfunctioning of the prostate would indicate that this theory is indeed true.

Is an enlarged prostate anything more than an enlarged muscle? Is an enlarged prostate not the sign of a virile, sexually active male?

Investigations reveal that the prostate is a muscle and increases in size as we mature. Some men have large solid arm muscles, for example, whereas others have large firm leg muscles or it could be that they have strong neck muscles or abdominal muscles.

In dealing with these muscles it must be recognized that many of these muscles can be seen or noticed when the person who has developed them wishes to show them. Then again, these specific muscles are the result of exercise or continued frequent use of that specific organ or part of the body.

Could the same principle not hold true with the prostate muscle? Does it not follow that by exercising the sexual organs of the body one will develop a strong, firm, hard or enlarged prostate?

Now the question that arises is this. Do acute retention of the urine and other symptoms always go hand in hand with an enlarged prostate? This is a question that needs to be answered ... but who is capable of answering it? So far I have encountered no one who is willing to accept the challenge and provide an answer to this perplexing problem. To the best of my knowledge, no research work has been done along these lines.

It is my belief that those men who do not participate actively in sexual relations have a normal or a small prostate gland. It is my further belief that the size of the prostate increases with the frequency of sexual relations until, due to sexual indulgence and over-indulgence, the prostate enlarges to the state where it eventually causes retention of the urine. Of course continued masturbation could produce the same result.

And then we are back again to the old bogey, "What is normal sexual frequency?" If we could find an answer to this enigma, we might then be closer to a solution for prostate disorders.

My studies indicate that disorders and diseases of the prostate are the most common and the most disturbing of all the conditions that affect adult males, and speaking from experience I would like to make this direct statement. Through the years of my life I have faced worries and troubles of many kinds and sorts, including financial, marital, familial as well as others to which most human beings are subject, but until I had trouble with my prostate, I must admit that I didn't know what worry really meant.

Now one authority, with whom I have been in contact, emphatically claims that there is a relationship between the womb and the prostate and states that the same embryonic tissue comprises both the womb and the prostate. The changes that take place in the prostate gland at middle age are very similar or practically identical to the changes that take place in the womb at the time of menopause.

It is definitely recognized that many men find they can't think as clearly and as straight as they used to and that their judgment and ability to concentrate have been affected. It is a fact that many business managers who should have and could have succeeded, because they possessed the inherent ability, failed because of the weakened judgment caused by prostate suffering.

There is no question about it, with the onset of prostate disorders a man's troubles increase and a man's ambition and drive decline. When a man is troubled with his prostate, for some reason he often becomes slow and sluggish and the old pep that was there seems to have dried up and disappeared. Work, tasks and chores that he once accepted gladly and willingly, and which he really enjoyed doing, are put off and delayed or not done at all.

Many a man has also become bitter and soured on things and his way of life and the world in general. His viewpoint becomes affected and he finds it difficult to find anything good or pleasant in people or life any more. He becomes peevish, fault-finding, fretful and even quarrelsome, whereas he was never like that when he was his usual self -- that is, before his prostate gave him trouble.

Then, too, his temper becomes short and, somewhat like a dog, he snaps frequently at people. This often happens among the folks he loves the best -- even at home, including his wife and children. Family, friends and associates who have known this person for a lifetime are unable to understand this drastic change in the individual.

I have found from my actual questioning that the disturbance resulting from the prostate does give a man more mental anguish than any other aspect of living. Over and over again I have come across individuals who were depressed, who were troubled and irritable, who were nervous and near exhaustion, who could not sleep, who did not know what to do with themselves, yet they could not lay the root of the trouble by the heels ... and in the majority of cases it was due to some malfunction of the prostate.

When you see this developing within yourself, it is time to do a bit of self-analysis or soul-searching. Stop and think and ask yourself, "Is my prostate giving me trouble? What is wrong with me?"

Therefore, it is my suggestion that prostate trouble can wear a thousand faces and can be the centre of turmoil where it is never suspected. Do not let a troublesome prostate ruin your life!

A friend of mine who is a highly intelligent, capable and learned physician, phrased it most succinctly when he said, "No man can be expected to think and act rationally in business or at home when he has trouble with his prostate."

I have been toying with the theory that prostatic hypertrophy is akin to or the same as goiter. While goiter is generally believed to be caused by deficiency of iodine in the human body, I would suggest that an enlarged prostate may be caused by deficiency of vitamin F.

The relationship between vitamin F and natural oil has not been definitely established but I believe vitamin F is found in all natural vegetable oils and animal fats. Adequate quantities of natural essential oils are found in all seeds in their raw, untreated condition. Some edible and palatable seeds that fit into this category are sunflower, sesame, flax, pumpkin and, of course, all nuts.

Our refined, synthetic, civilized way of preparing foods kills the vitamin F or makes it unavailable to the body by the various treatments, including heat, refinement or chemicalization. The prostate gland enlarges in an effort to protect itself and improve its functions, which, next to those of the heart, are the most important functions of the human body ... one of which is the carrying of the seminal fluid for procreation.

It is important to note that neglect of enlargement of the prostate gland can and often does cause disease of the kidneys. The too frequent need for bladder emptying and the general resulting starting and stopping of urination, often culminates in dribbling. I warn that permitting such a situation to continue can in the long run lead to serious trouble. If this condition is neglected over a long period of time the destruction of kidney tissue may be the end result.

Then eventually, if no positive action is taken, there comes a time when retention of the urine occurs -- complete blockage. At such time, if relief is not found, the urine backs up and this can cause serious, often irreparable kidney injury. Just how many of the kidney diseases are due to trouble with the prostate has never been established but you can be sure that it is one, if not the chief cause of kidney disease. Therefore, it is not wise to allow prostate troubles to continue without some attempt at correcting the condition. It is wise, when there is threat of such disorders, to promptly contact a qualified practitioner.

One of the vital things to be concerned about in latent prostatism without residual urine is that it may remain unrecognized for a long period and be harmless except in so far as the tendency to the development of carcinoma may be increased by it. However, as soon as residual urine has developed, the kidney function becomes more or less impaired and the cardio-vascular system is involved secondarily. The course is progressive and complete retention develops in time. Other things being equal, the longer the time between the development of residual urine and of complete retention the greater the damage of the renal function.

It is generally established and understood that cancer of the prostate is considered the least progressive in growth of any of the cancers, but once cancer of the prostate is diagnosed it is regarded as a most serious condition. I am quoting from a most authoritative medical journal which says:

"Conservative urologists of many years of experience defer operation until they are definitely certain that there is some progression. It must be remembered that this is a very serious operation, the mortality is high, and the possibility of stirring up trouble and sending some of the cancer cells from the prostate into a remote organ is not too small. Death then occurs in a few months."

An accepted medical authority on the prostate claims that 18% to 20% of the prostate overgrowths are due to cancer and the symptoms are practically the same as those of simple enlargement.

One authority states that the development of prostatic hypertrophy and even cancer of the gland are caused by the hormonal efforts of the testicles and other reproductive glands as well as the adrenals to keep the procreational abilities functioning and alive. He contends that as a result of the increase in the male sex hormones the prostatic tissues are stimulated and thus grow.

Due to this condition the lobes increase greatly in size and form a dam at the neck of the bladder. This prevents complete emptying of the bladder. With continued activation, followed by growth and more obstruction, the bladder loses its capacity to empty its contents thoroughly and completely -- with the result that the patient must urinate frequently. This is more noticeable during the night because it interferes with proper rest and sleep.

Prostatism is a general clinical term which may be conveniently used to include all of the disturbances to urination induced by obstruction of any sort occurring at the neck. The anatomical lesions producing these changes are adenoma (hypertrophy), carcinoma and fibrosis (sclerosis of the prostate, contracture of the bladder neck, etc.) of the prostate or in the prostatic urethra. Some prostatic disorders are (1) acute prostatitis, (2) chronic prostatitis, (3) hemorrhagic prostatitis, (4) hypertrophy of the prostate, (5) atrophy of the prostate, (6) non-specific prostatitis.

Chapter Three

SYMPTOMS

How is one to recognize the signs of prostate troubles? Is it to be assumed that all genital malfunctions or urinary difficulties are afflictions of the prostate?

It is no exaggeration to say that there are so many signs and conditions that might indicate prostatic troubles that I could easily devote half the book to the discussion of these symptoms alone. It is my belief that many of the symptoms that are attributed to the prostate have no connection with the prostate whatsoever. Among certain practitioners, whenever a man past 40 comes to them for advice and claims to have occasional or frequent backaches, the prostate is the number one suspect.

Trying to pinpoint symptoms that indicate trouble a-brewing with the prostate is indeed a major undertaking. A great deal of time was expended in study and investigation, gathering the data that is contained in this chapter. Then there was also my personal experience and travail.

While it is admitted that one might have

many genital derangements that have no root or connection with the prostate, yet I would go on record as advising caution and suspicion with any malfunction that originates in the area surrounding the genital organs. I strongly advise that when such conditions arise, look to the prostate.

Now I will give you a list of conditions, symptoms or signs that may indicate trouble with the prostate:

1. Pains between the legs and in the rectum.
2. Pains and a burning sensation in the urethra and penis.
3. Pains in the lower back or hip or groin.
4. Chronic constipation along with the feeling that there is a lump in the rectum.
5. Feeling the need to evacuate the bowel but being unable to do so.
6. Difficulty in starting urination, thinness of stream with dribbling at the end.
7. Leakage of urine.
8. A discharge from the urethra.
9. Nervous irritability along with a feeling of depression or melancholia.
10. Frequent urination along with improper emptying of the bladder.
11. A burning sensation of the feet.
12. Pains in the back of the neck at the base of the skull.
13. Frequent urination during the night.
14. Disturbed sleep.

15. A piercing, painful or burning feeling during urination.
16. Slackening of sexual vigor.
17. Lessening of sexual satisfaction.
18. Difficulty in maintaining an erection.
19. Cloudy color in the urine, indicating mucous from the prostate is passing out of the urethra.
20. Tightening sensation in the testes.
21. Pains of a severe nature in the testes.
22. Lack of energy and a general feeling of tiredness.
23. Numb feeling in the crotch or at the base of the genital organs.
24. Unexplainable headaches.
25. Inability to concentrate in a normal manner.

The most definite and recognizable indication that there is something wrong with the prostate is discomfort in passing urine. If these warnings are neglected for an extended period, you may one day be confronted by a definite blockage or retention. However when you have reached the latter stage you are almost invariably in for trouble, varying from bad to serious. I hope that you who are reading this book will not wait until you have retention of the urine before you realize that something is amiss.

Of course, there can be retention of the urine without actually involving any prostatic malfunction, but such situations are extremely rare. If you went to a practitioner and complained about urinary disorders or malfunctions of the genitals, one of the first things he would do would be to make a digital rectal examination. This is done by inserting a prepared finger into the rectum. In this way the practitioner can readily feel the prostate gland. This, of course, would only indicate whether or not the prostate was enlarged.

One of the early signs of prostate trouble is frequent urination ... but of course, this can also occur when diabetes is involved. Actually very few men complain of frequent urination in the early stages, and for a very good reason. They are loathe to admit this sign of physical degeneration even to themselves. They believe or have been told that this is just a sign of advancing age and when this happens to them when they get to be around 50 or 60, they are conditioned to expect it without actually accepting it. However, age has little or nothing to do with the frequency of urination when the body and glands are functioning properly. For example, I know many men in their seventies who do not have frequent urination.

Often in the earlier stages of prostate derangement, the patient complains of a dull, aching pain in the nape of the neck right up close to the skull, usually more to the left side than the right. This pain can become quite severe and frequently medical men prescribe and advise the use of some form of pain reliever which tends to mask the source of the disorder. I would suggest that you be very suspicious of pains emanating from the base of the skull.

The feeling that the bladder is never completely empty, no matter how frequently one urinates, is a more or less definite indication that prostate trouble exists.

Any strange aches or twinges around the groin area or pains that linger around the lower back and the upper parts of the legs are often indicative of prostate trouble.

Many men will complain of feelings of depression and melancholia and when this comes with a loss of sexual drive, some authorities feel this is the male change of life or as it is sometimes called, 'the male climacteric.' However, this could also indicate something amiss with the prostate.

When a normal, seemingly healthy man who is accustomed to regular sexual relations starts to slip sexually, I would advise a period of profound thinking coupled with the reading and studying of sound unprejudiced health literature or a consultation with a professional healer.

Marked lessening of one's sexual desires, the inability to properly perform the sex act, the inability to maintain an erection or the lack of interest in female friends could indicate a disturbance of the prostate.

Men with serious prostate difficulties no longer find a pair of trim ankles and a shapely figure attractive and alluring ... and slowly the usual joys and pleasures of living seem to wane. It is my belief that if this condition is permitted to continue, senility will be the end result.

Often the suspicion of being afflicted

with a prostatic disorder will make men practise self-denial and they seek to avoid sexual relations. Then in many cases there lies the fear that they will be unable to complete the act and thus be humiliated. To save themselves shame and embarrassment and to avoid a discontented, unsatisfied mate, they put off the act and claim indisposition, debility or illness ... or offer some other lame excuse.

The longer the signs of a deteriorating prostate are ignored and the condition is tolerated, and the longer the individual goes without sexual relationship, the greater the threat to his health and the more the condition is being seriously aggravated.

It is an established fact that one who indulges in regular sexual intercourse tends to require and desire it more frequently than one who indulges but rarely. It is simply a matter of logic ... the more sexual intercourse you have, the more you need and the more you want. By the same token, the less you have the less you want and need.

This axiom is one that is absolutely true. Anyone with wide experience in matters pertaining to sexual activity knows that a sexually vigorous young man has a tendency to be a sexually vigorous old man and one who has infulged only rarely in sexual relations when young tends to indulge even less when he gets older. A muscle or an organ that is used frequently remains in a condition to be used frequently and an organ that is neglected and unused eventually atrophies and can hardly be used at all.

This is simple arithmetic.

I consider sexual disorders or impairment a strong indication that something is amiss with the prostate and therefore, when you are facing any one of the many predicaments that may arise with your sex organs or sexual relations, I would certainly look to the prostate.

No one can gainsay the importance of sustained sexual potency to the male of the species and a properly functioning prostate is essential for sexual potency.

Often anxiety, worry and a vivid imagination play havoc with a man's libido. While on occasion such a situation can be strictly psychosomatic, yet a failing prostate can be the direct cause of such behaviours.

Sometimes the appearance of a thin, mucous-like, oily substance which trickles from the urethra without sexual stimulation or provocation is another indication that all is not well with the prostate. This fluid is the prostate gland secretion and even a mild sustained flow of this substance, unless accompanied by sexual excitement, is known as prostatorrhea. It is believed that this condition is often brought about by fear and worry.

Often when men see the escaping fluid they believe it is seminal fluid and are frightened, for they think their very life's blood is ebbing away.

This condition may also be caused by inflammation of the Cowperian glands, known as Cowperites, but very little is known about this condition or even about the Cowperian glands, commonly called Cowper's glands. One authority suggests that they produce an alkaline secretion that acts to neutralize an acidity that might inhibit the activity and flow of the spermatozoa.

When things go wrong with normal ejaculation, this indicates that the seminal vesicles and the prostate gland are in a state of hyper-excitability. Sometimes the ejaculation is painful or late or even premature. Occasionally signs of blood are noticed in the ejaculation or an ejaculation occurs without sexual excitement or without any feeling that an ejaculation is taking place. These, too, are signs that something is amiss with the prostate.

There is no denying that there may be other signs, indications or manifestations of a degenerating prostate but they did not turn up in my serious probings. However, to the best of my knowledge, no one individual or organization has ever made any serious attempt to find the cause of most diseases ... so why should we expect anyone to do so for prostate disease? Who cares about causes? There is no money or glory in that field but there is a "Fort Knox" in cures, nostrums and surgery!

Chapter Four

IS PROSTATE TROUBLE A DISEASE OF OLD AGE?

From the information I have been able to gather from medical doctors, chiropractors, naturopaths, medical herbalists, homeopathic doctors, osteopaths and other healers, it was for a long time generally accepted and believed that disease of the prostate was an old man's disease. The reason? For many years 75% of the men over 70 years of age have had prostate troubles of one kind or another.

Similarly we could say that cancer is a disease of old age because most of the people who get cancer are old. And there is little doubt about it, if you live long enough, you will more than likely become heir to prostate trouble, a heart attack, cancer or any one of the other degenerative diseases.

It is a fact, from statistical figures supplied to me, that diseases of the prostate cause approximately 20,000 deaths (1962 figures) each year in the United States alone ... and this toll appears to be increasing steadily. By the year 1968 this toll is expected to reach 25,000 deaths each year from various prostate conditions.

It is estimated that at least 75% of the 20,000 deaths are attributed to cancer of the prostate.

Prostatic conditions are among the most important of all ailments for which men aged 65 and over seek medical care. Estimates clearly indicate that the population of men aged 65 and over in the United States will increase by 500,000 within the next five years ... which will bring this total to approximately 8,350,000 who are over 65 years of age in the United States.

It is my solemn prediction that prostatic conditions will continue to increase steadily. Thus a much greater amount of space will be required in hospitals to provide care for men suffering from various prostatic diseases.

Nowhere has anyone made any attempt to discover the causative factors. It would appear as though prostatic disease is accepted or believed to be a disease of advancing age and therefore it is felt that nothing need be or can be done.

I maintain most stoutly that there are causative factors and that these causative factors could be found or isolated if research was undertaken. In fact, I have enumerated what I believe to be the most important causative factors of prostate disorders ... and when at last the true cause or causes are found, I predict that my thesis will be found to be on solid ground.

It should be stressed that frequent urination and nocturnal urination are positively not due to old age or natural conditions. Furthermore, both conditions are not always caused by an enlarged prostate.

I realize that it is widely accepted and often taught by healers that both these conditions prove that the prostate is enlarged but I emphatically insist that this is not always true. Yes, an enlarged prostate can cause urinary frequency, brought about by the bladder being dammed by a greatly enlarged prostate, yet it is not always the case.

The time-worn argument of apologists for the status quo group would, of course, have us believe that due to the great advances in chemistry, hygiene, medicine, surgery and the social services, we now live longer and more people reach old age ... and thus, more live to have prostate trouble.

But this argument is ruled out in this case, for now, in this present day and age, prostate disorders are quite common in men from 30 years of age upwards ... and the number is increasing rapidly! However, it is granted that the older the age group the higher the incidence of prostate trouble. Then again, it has been stated that you are as old as your prostate!

There isn't the faintest doubt in my mind that at the turn of the century or prior, disease of the prostate was definitely an old man's disease. However, for some strange reason, which no one at the present time is definitely able to explain, prostate troubles are being encountered quite frequently in young men ... and at middle age it is widespread. This would point directly at our mode of living, for no one can deny that we in America, especially, have changed our way of life drastically in the past 50 years.

Statistics are funny things. Some people place great store in them and others, like myself, sort of shrug and say, "Well, that's what it says -- just what does it mean?"

However, here I would like to quote statistics and estimates concerning the incidence of prostate troubles among men, so you will get some idea as to what the various experts, authorities and writers have found or believe. You will see that there is a great variation in the figures given but one thing will come up stark and clear ... and that is that prostate troubles are part and parcel of the life of practically every male beyond the age of 50.

Here are some of the figures given:

40% of all men beyond the age of 60 have prostate troubles
66 2/3% of all men beyond the age of 60
65% of all men beyond 50
65% of all men past 50 have enlargement of the prostate
20% of these enlargements become malignant
60% of all men past 40 have prostate troubles
90% of all males over 50 have prostate trouble
20% of all males over 40 have cancer of the prostate
80% of men have gonorrhea some time

in life

65% of all men between the ages of 60 and 70 have prostate hypertrophy or hyperplasia

More men over 65 years of age suffer from prostate conditions than from any other single disease or malfunction

Practically all men will develop an enlarged prostate if they live long enough

I have consulted as many doctors as I could find who had lived in and had experience in the East. In every case, without exception, these doctors told me that they seldom ran across anyone with prostate trouble.

One doctor said, "I practised medicine in China for twenty-odd years and during that time did not observe many patients complaining of symptoms that would suggest prostate trouble. I practised in China proper just in the vicinity of the Yellow River in Honan province adjoining Shantung province on the eastern coast and so well to the east of the country as a whole."

Another doctor who practised in Burma told me that he did not encounter any prostate troubles and the reason he gave was that he felt that most natives didn't live to be old enough to have prostate troubles.

However, it is a fact that these doctors who each spent 20 or more years in the East, seldom, if ever, ran across patients who were suffering from prostate troubles.

One of the difficulties in dealing with prostate disorders is the fact that most men are shy or reluctant to reveal that they are suffering from a prostate disorder. They tend to hide their troubles because they seem to think it is a reflection upon their sexual abilities or their way of life. You will often find men even trying to hide this condition from their wives, fearing that it will cause their wives to look down upon them or fearful lest their wives think of them as being "over the hill."

The plain truth is, if a man will face up to the situation and recognize that he is encountering a serious condition that requires early analysis and treatment, the sooner his condition can be remedied or completely eradicated and prevent the so-called trail "over the hill." However, ignoring the truth and trying to hide it can spell disaster to what has been up until then a happy marriage. Furthermore, seeking to hide the true condition often affects a man's mental outlook and does harm or interferes with his work or his business activities.

One rather interesting and probably valid thesis promulgated by a capable naturopathic physician claims that when a male gets beyond 40 his testicles become less active and shrink and as a compensatory measure, his prostate enlarges.

Another brilliant doctor claims that no organ in the human body can properly function without the stimulating aid of the internal secretion from the sex gland -- referring specifically to the prostate gland.

Anyone knows that castrated animals seldom ever live as long as normal unscathed animals. Seldom if ever does a eunuch attain the age of 65. Of course there are cases, due to prostate cancer and such, where men have been emasculated at 70 and 75 and even 80. I am citing this to indicate that therefore there are older emasculated men.

I am acquainted with and have talked to many men and among them are some who are my friends, none of whom are old men (not over 65) and there are a goodly number of them, who, for any one of many reasons, no longer partake of or enjoy sexual activity. Therefore I know it is true. Invariably those who no longer enjoy sex have lost their lust for life in all its facets, as well as their zest and joy of living. I suspect that many religious zealots fit neatly into this category.

Therefore, it is vitally important that every man do all within his power to retain his sexual virility and to protect his prostate because he needs it, as I have outlined.

I recall that I heard of prostate surgery occasionally when I was a youth 40 or 50 years ago. In those days surgical techniques in general, but especially for prostate surgery, were quite primitive, extremely painful and the mortality rate was very high. My father had prostate trouble and I recall that at least half a dozen of his close friends and associates had prostate surgery. Furthermore, I was well acquainted not only with their troubles but with the agony and suffering which they underwent after surgery, which was done in two operations.

However, the men mentioned above were all in their middle 60's and some their 70's. Today among my friends and associates in their 50's it is quite prevalent and many men in their 40's and some in their 30's have indicated that there is something wrong with their urinary or plumbing system, as I call it.

To prove or disprove my contention that it is now becoming prevalent among the young men, the next time you enter a public lavatory, note how many of the men step up smartly to the urinal, perform the needed function and then without much fussing, step away. You'll be surprised when most of them step up, remain standing for 10, 20, 30 seconds -- sometimes a minute -- before the flow starts. When the flow has subsided, then starts the shut-off and drip and the maneuvering to get rid of the last insistent drops. All this, let me say to you, is a positive indication of the beginning of prostate trouble. I sincerely suggest that you make this test.

Back before World War I in 1910 or 1911, J. H. Tilden in his writing stated that seldom was an older man found who did not have some urinary problems such as are today considered indicative of prostate disorders.

Here is a quotation from E. Shaftesbury, M.D., regarding the use of one of our most popular beverages:

"Beware of Tea. Tea enjoys the pleasant status of being a poisoner. To be sure, the United States Government in a bulletin announced iced tea as slow suicide. One cup does no perceptible harm; yet the heart and vital centers have been hurt some small fraction of one per cent, and will never again be just as sound. It requires years before the heart gets leaky, the liver stale, the kidneys sluggish, the lungs weak and the stomach flabby; but they get there just the same.

"The bladder is about the first organ to furnish evidence of the damage from quieting the nerves. The contents of the bladder are held in place by a certain valve that opens only when the mind orders, although some young folks have not the power to control it, especially during sleep. This valve is dependent on the energy of the nerves to hold it shut. After years of having the nerves quietened by tea-drinking, they are no longer able to keep the bladder valve shut tight. It opens, and the water of the bladder drops out and saturates the clothing.

"Have you ever entered the room of a house where tea-drinking women and old men are assembled and noticed as you came in from outdoors the close and deadening smell of dropped urine? Even young folks afford this odour if they are tea-drinkers to quieten their nerves to any extent. There is not an old codger living today who does not wear clothing saturated with this odour if he has been a tea-drinker; and there is not an old man tea-drinker with a sound bladder valve. Tea-drinking women overload themselves with perfumes to conceal the real state of their bladder trouble, but the concealment is never complete."

Today the counterpart can be found in beverage rooms, bars, cocktail lounges, 'pubs' and other places where alcoholic beverage drinkers congregate.

Let us ask ourselves a pertinent question. If prostate trouble once was considered a disease of old age, why has it now become a disease that affects young and middle-aged men? It is vitally important that we study the situation and examine our way of life so that we may learn the causative factors and find a way to avoid them.

Chapter Five

WHAT IS RETENTION?

An accumulation of urine in the bladder for a considerable period, at least something beyond 12 hours, is usually recognized as retention or stoppage of the urine.

There are many causes of retention of the urine. Retention sometimes follows an obstruction from disease, along with a temporary swelling and nervous contraction of some part of the uro-genital passage. It may be caused by spasms and closure of the outlet or from injuries and surgical operations in the vicinity of the sexual organs or the rectum. It can also be caused by tumors of the urinary tract or adjacent organs such as the prostate. On occasions stones or strictures, either in the lower or upper portions of the canal, will cause obstructions. Then, too, various general physical disorders such as severe fevers, unconsciousness and other disorders of the nervous system, can be accompanied by retention of the urine. Hysteria may also cause retention.

A top-ranking healer states that acute

retention of the urine may be brought about by chills or heavy drinking, alone or in combination. Such things can cause the already enlarged prostate gland to swell even further, thus damming off or blocking the flow of urine. When retention does strike, great pain is suffered by the affected individual.

Acute retention is often suffered by men who have gone on hunting or other sporting expeditions and have become exposed to the elements for extended periods, such as sitting on cold rocks or in damp locations. This, coupled with perspiration brought on by previous effort, can cause acute retention.

Now I want to describe another most unusual and important change that takes place. As the enlarged prostate expands upwards it also affects the position and elasticity of the bladder and at the same time stretches the urethra lengthwise like a narrow rubber tube, to the extent that it almost closes the passage ... often completely causing a shut-off.

Now let us examine the illustrations facing Page 51. They show the genito-urinary organs, a section of the mouth of the urethra, an enlarged prostate and a normal prostate. In the first illustration you will see the position of the normal prostate in relation to the bladder and the urethra. In the second illustration you can see the enlarged prostate gland forcing the bladder out of its normal functioning position.

You will note that as the prostate enlarges upward it heaves the bladder out of shape, which actually reduces the carrying capacity of the bladder as well as forming a dam behind which residual urine remains almost continuously. This "damming off" of urine in the bladder is the reason why those who have prostate trouble feel as though the bladder is never empty. It may also be a contributing factor in dribbling and post-urinal drip. This damming of the bladder also tends to partially cut off the flow of urine.

This condition may also cause cystitis which is described as "inflammation of the bladder with pus and blood." This may cause serious trouble with the kidneys.

One specialist relates that the symptoms of simple overgrowth, enlargement or as it is technically called, hypertrophy, and the symptoms of cancer of the prostate are identical. He suggests that prostate disease can be treated by administering the female sex hormones to neutralize the stimulating influence of the male hormones and that cortisone will at times delay progress of the disease by its action on the androgen (male sex hormones) producing adrenal. He urges surgery where required, stating that prostate surgery does not necessarily mean the loss of sexual ability. He stresses the fact that the danger of kidney and heart damage becomes progressively worse as the obstruction progresses and the unfounded fears of impotency should not delay needed surgery.

The term "stricture" as used in referring to prostate difficulty indicates that it is a morbid narrowing of a canal, a passage or a duct. This term is generally used in referring to the urethra but it could also refer to the esophagus or the intestine. It is suggested by some authorities that a stricture is brought about by an overgrowth of the prostate extending, spreading or creeping over into the urethra -- slowly but surely -- and eventually it winds up blocking the passage.

Incontinence of Urine: By incontinence is meant the involuntary passage of urine from the bladder. It is classified as false (paradoxical) if it occurs in the presence of a distended bladder and as true if the bladder holds little or no urine. Complete incontinence, in which no urine at all is held in the bladder is rare: incomplete incontinence the rule.

Marked distention produces sufficient pressure on the impaired muscle to force it so that some urine passes, but not sufficient to empty the bladder. The dribbling of urine after urination in advanced stricture cases is often due to impaired action of the bulbo and ischio-cavernosis muscles and is not a real incontinence.

1. False (paradoxical) incontinence. Occurs in chronic retention from:

   (a) Prostatism.
   (b) Urethral stricture.
   (c) Nervous diseases, such as tabes, myelitis, transverse cord lesions, etc.

2. True incontinence. Occurs:

(a) In bladder fistulae. Some urine maybe retained and normal urination be possible if the fistulae in small. It is due to birth injuries, operations, or accidents. Incontinence of this type may be simulated by abnormal opening of the ureters into the urethra.

(b) In lesions of the bladder neck and sphincter due to:
   (1) Inflammation (tuberculosis of bladder or prostate).
   (2) Infiltration by neoplasm.

(c) In weakening of bladder sphincters:
   (1) In diseases of the nervous system.
   (2) From stretching the sphincter mechanically.
   (3) Inactivity.

(d) Interference with normal closing of bladder sphincter by:
   (1) Impacted stones.
   (2) Tumors (movable or pedunculated).
   (3) Hyperirritability of detrusor
   (4) Incoordination of sphincter and detrusor, (eneuresis, epilepsy).

Treatment in false incontinence is that of chronic incomplete retention: in true incontinence that of the underlying disease.

The actual retention is seldom if ever

an accident that occurs on the spur of the moment. In practically every case it is brought about by various conditions that may date back years and, yes, even decades.

You could take any one of the causative factors that we have mentioned in another chapter or you could take some of them and sometimes even all of them and these taking place or occurring through 10, 20, 30, 40 or 50 years of life eventually cause a complete stoppage of the flow of urine.

It is claimed that the process actually starts with the swelling of the smallest sac-like dilations which compose the prostate gland. This swelling is due to the retention of the secretions which normally should be evacuated by sexual intercourse through the ejaculatory ducts in the process of intercourse. When this ejaculation does not occur because of any one of many reasons, the secretion becomes thicker and this leads to what the medical fraternity refers to as an infection, such as pus and inflammatory products that accumulate. If in due course these accumulations do not escape, cysts are formed. By means of the formation of these cysts and their progression in the prostate, the entire gland tends to enlarge. Various kinds, and too frequently the wrong kind, of bacterial action develop because everything is in favor of their development. Thus this continued action stimulates further swelling and enlargement of the gland, and the fibrous tissues enlarge and increase throughout the whole glandular structure.

If you will examine the diagram facing

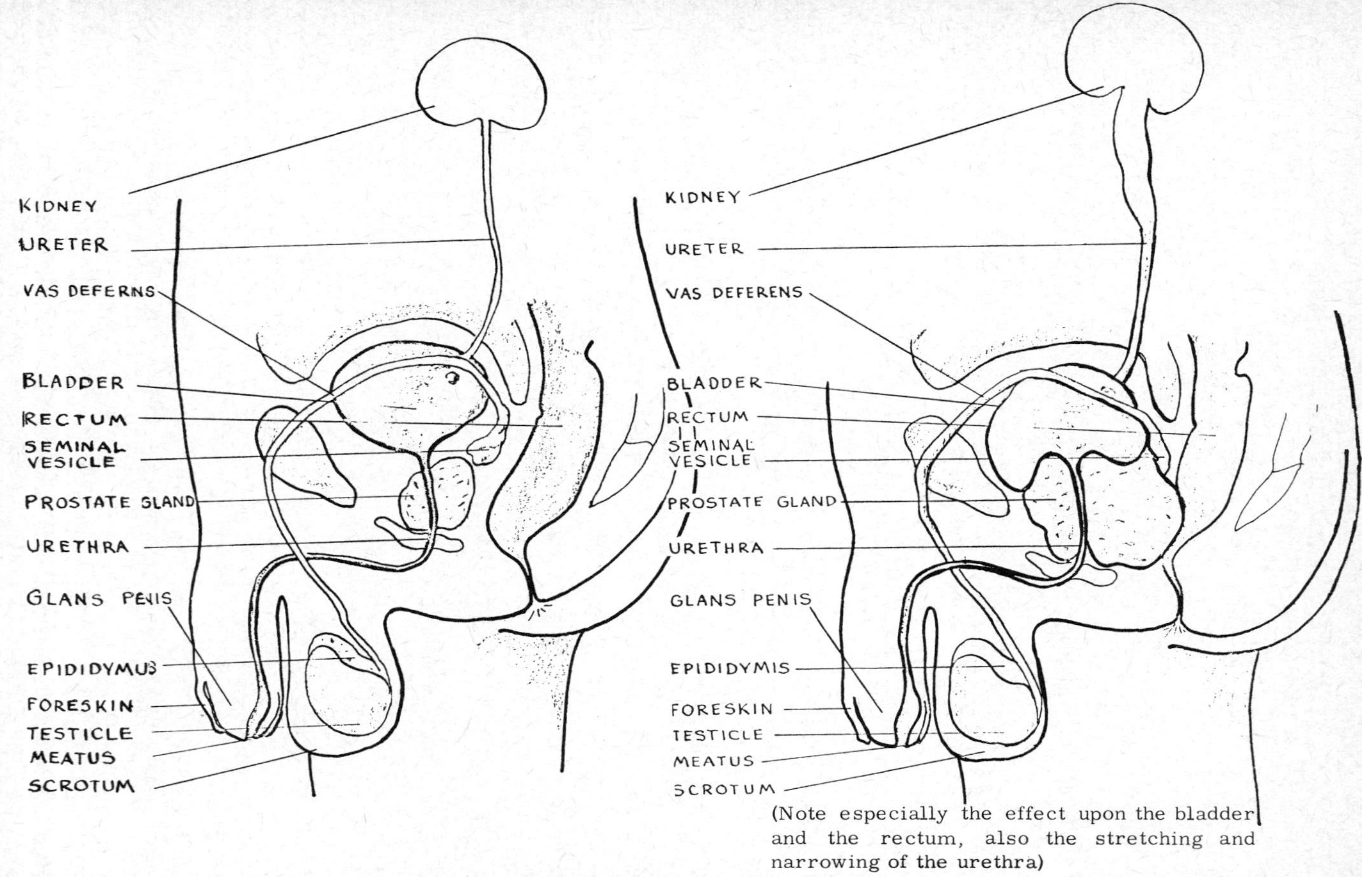

(Note especially the effect upon the bladder and the rectum, also the stretching and narrowing of the urethra)

Page 51 you will see that as the gland becomes enlarged it presses with considerable force into the rectum and then up into the bladder. This action will of course interfere with normal bowel movement and will broaden or sort of create a platform at the bottom of the bladder. As the urethral opening and the sphincter muscles are located at the bottom or the floor of the bladder, this means that the urethra is stretched upwards and its length is increased. The consequence is that while the length is increased, the channel is narrowed. This simply means that the whole urethra becomes longer and narrower. Thus, you can understand that the neck of the bladder and the prostatic urethra are forced out of their normal alinement and a sort of deformation takes place.

As this condition progresses it causes frequent urination because there are various dams formed and the best way I can explain this is by taking a rubber bottle -- for example, an ordinary hot water bottle. Turn it upside down and remove the stopper and the water will flow out freely. But if you force the neck of the water bottle upwards, then a certain amount of the fluid will not flow out ... and the higher up the opening of the bottle is forced, the more will be retained. Thus, there is a continued residue which in time causes irritation in the bladder. That is why you will often find that people who have allowed this condition to progress will urinate ten, fifteen or even twenty times a day. Then they will parade to the bathroom practically every hour on the hour during the night. When this condition is permitted to go on without a change in living habits or some other corrective measure, there comes a time when, because of a combination of the swelling of the prostate both inwards and outwards, the damming of the bladder and the stretching of the urethra, a complete retention occurs.

Basically this is all brought about due to the swelling or enlargement or engorgement or, as it is properly called, hypertrophy of the prostate gland. Therefore, the solution is to do whatever has to be done to prevent the prostate from swelling to that great size or to do what is necessary to reduce the swelling to permit the normal flow of urine.

The idea or suggestion of stooping on all fours like an animal to urinate is advice that has been given to many men who were suffering from prostate conditions or incomplete retention of the urine. The reason behind this maneuver is well founded for it is believed that it does actually tip the bladder so that it will have a better chance of emptying. This is because, as it is known, an enlarged overgrown prostate pushes upward into the bladder -- thus forming a dam which prevents the urine from draining properly.

Now mind you, this does sound a bit troublesome but from the reports that I've had from those who have practised it, they do definitely get improved micturition and thus, less residual urine is left in the bladder. This exercise is usually practised before retiring for the night.

Here is an interesting reference to the prostate condition from a book published in 1908. I think it is well done and I am quoting it . . .

"Except in very few instances in which a sudden retention of the urine is the first indication of an enlarged prostate, the time which elapses from the appearance of the earliest and usually slight symptoms to those which are alarming is ordinarily a long one; it is quite common for it to extend over two or three years, frequently it covers five or six, and not rarely eight or ten. In spite of its slow development the disease never stands still, never retrogrades and never subsides without good care. Therefore, an almost imperceptible advance in the gravity of one's experiences is not an indication that serious trouble will not ensue finally. He who allows matters to go so far that retention occurs, 'catheter life' has to be entered upon, or cystitis or stone develops, courts disaster and puts himself in a position from which he may be rescued with difficulty."

Here is another phrasing of this condition in more technical language:

"The effect of prostatic enlargement is to obstruct the out-flow of urine. Enlargement of the lateral lobes compresses the urethra into a narrow and irregular slit. Enlargement of the median lobe or the subcervical glands of Albarran results in a nodular mass which pushes up the floor of the bladder just inside the sphincter or in proximal part of the urethra. This midline enlargement is particularly effective in obstructing outflow of urine, acting as a plug to close the urethral orifice. A small sac forms behind the prostatic nodule, from which urine cannot be expelled, and contains the so-called residual urine."

It is quite possible that other factors may play a role in retention but the facts illustrated in this chapter are usually recognized and accepted.

Chapter Six

CAUSES OF PROSTATE DISORDERS

Section A -- Consensus of Opinion

I have searched through mountains of literature, I have studied countless case histories, I have questioned hundreds of sufferers, and this I can tell you with some degree of authority ... there is no known single, definite cause of prostate disorders.

One of the best known and most widely recognized authorities in the medical field says of enlarged prostate gland: "The actual cause of this condition is unknown. It is especially likely to occur in men who have frequent inflammation of the prostate in early life. Enlarged prostate is a true tumoral formation and a certain percentage becomes cancerous."

Therefore, from this statement and the testimony and writings of other authorities, it would be broadly recognized that in their opinion there is no positive known cause of enlarged prostate.

During the time I was preparing this work on the prostate I consulted innumerable healers, covering all of the healing arts, and in every case I asked them if they knew the cause of prostate disorders. While many of them hazarded guesses and gave their opinions, not one of them would definitely state that any one specific factor was the cause or would bring about disease of the prostate.

Alcohol

Of course many of them suggested some of the same things. For example, in practically every case the use of alcohol was mentioned as one of the causes.

I do not specifically claim that alcohol is the cause of prostate trouble but I do know for an absolute certainty that the use of alcohol can irritate or cause a latent condition to flare up and suddenly become acute. My questioning has revealed that every authority will attest to this fact. Then, of course, many of them blame the use of alcohol as one of the most important causative factors. The difference is that I do not specifically blame alcohol as a causative factor ... but I do know for certain that it frequently triggers the condition.

It is also my belief that highly seasoned foods and spices act in a similar manner ... that is, they are not the basic causative factors but will irritate a condition that already exists.

Many healers blamed the following: coffee drinking, tea drinking, smoking, overindulgence in sex, masturbation, venereal diseases, delay in answering nature's call, sedentary occupations, long trips in motor cars, and many other hypotheses.

On the other hand, I have found men who did not smoke or drink or use coffee or tea, who did not have gonorrhea or syphilis or commit any of the other violations mentioned, yet they had prostate trouble.

One volume gave these causes: Gonorrhea, stricture of the urethra, cystitis, stone in the bladder, sexual over-indulgence, masturbation, excessive horseback or bicycle riding, alcoholic intemperance, a sedentary life, and making a practice of holding the urine for long periods.

There is no doubt about it ... the disease often develops in those who, to all appearances and to the best information that I could gather about them, have led a blameless and model life in every respect and have never previously had any affliction of the urinary organs.

The foregoing statement is stressed because it actually does happen that even if all the normal conventional rules of living and health are followed, prostate infection still occurs.

Coffee

A friend of mine -- a biochemist, highly esteemed in his profession and whom I consider one of the best versed men on foods and chemicals -- informs me that in his opinion coffee is an important contributor to prostate disorders and he gives the following reasons: (a) Because of the volatile oils that are freed by the treatments in making the coffee, (b) Due to the carcinogenic factors caused by roasting or burning, (c) Due to the various chemicals that are added in the processing of or in the canning, (d) The burning sensation often found when urinating is caused by an over-dose of caffeine.

It is widely accepted by all of the healing arts that there are a host of contributing factors, but as yet no one single factor has been discovered which positively causes any one of the many prostate disorders. Yet, it is recognized that a great number of things -- actions, conditions, deeds, habits and circumstances -- are suspect ... but as of the time that I am writing, I must repeat, no positive cause has been established.

Obesity

Dr. Tilden claims, "My experience has been that stout men, or men with heavy abdomens, are more liable to prostate enlargement than are men of slender build, due to the pressure of the heavy abdomen on the pelvic organs."

It is claimed that acute prostatitis may develop during the course of the following diseases: small pox, scarlet fever, typhoid fever and typhus.

Hardening of the Arteries

Then someone else maintains that hardening of the arteries and enlargement of the prostate appear to be related. It seems that anyone who has hardening of the arteries usually has an enlarged prostate and anyone who has an enlarged prostate usually has hardening of the arteries.

Smoking

Some authorities claim that smoking is a causative factor in prostate diseases. I definitely do not go along on this theory because I know too many men who do not smoke -- never did smoke -- and yet have prostate trouble.

Venereal Diseases

Many men are afraid to admit that they have prostate trouble because they have been told that prostate troubles are the result of venereal infection. Again I want to emphasize that this is absolutely not true.

While gonorrhea is frequently blamed as being a cause of prostatic disease, my investigations positively reveal that most of the prostate troubles are definitely not caused by gonorrhea or any other form of venereal disease. I wish to emphasize this fact because statistical studies clearly indicate that more men are troubled with prostatic enlargement who have never had gonorrhea than those who have suffered with this culpable disease. Further, I am led to believe that if it is the onslaught of gonorrhea, then it is the treatment and the drugs that are administered for this disease that cause the prostate trouble and not the disease itself.

Furthermore, as quoted elsewhere in this book, a respected and knowledgeable physician wrote to me and informed me that one of the easiest ways to avoid prostate troubles is to have venereal disease when you are young because somehow it seems to bring about a condition that means you will not have prostate trouble when you grow older. So you can see that medical opinion is somewhat divided or hazy on the subject!

Now while the doctor who gave me that suggestion about the venereal diseases was serious when he wrote it to me, I still would certainly frown upon this type of advice. Even though, as he claims "it seems to bring about a condition that means you will not have prostate trouble when you grow older," yet I think prostate diseases would not be as bad or as harmful as the condition brought about by the venereal disease.

At first I had qualms about quoting this piece about venereal diseases and the advice given me by this highly respected physician, but I felt that as I was trying to get all the information possible into my book, I wanted to leave no stones unturned.

While it would be comparatively simple and most useful to blame "germs," "infections," and "viruses" for prostatic disease, rational thinking and common sense indicate that it is, in truth, none of these most useful healers' scapegoats but the violation of biological principles that bring on the trouble.

I have also read reports where sexual indulgence during menstruation has been blamed as a causative factor in prostate diseases. I realize that no one can positively and emphatically state that this could not be a contributor, but I, for one, will not accept this as a legitimate influence.

Dental Factors

One authority has mentioned decayed, caried, abscessed teeth or pus pockets in the tonsils as being causes of prostatic disorders.

Systemic Diseases

It has further been suggested that some of the systemic diseases like typhoid, influenza and malaria might also cause malfunctions of the prostate and one well known practitioner claimed that a typhoid infection caused one of the largest infected prostate that he had ever seen. This same practitioner insinuates that leucorrhea or "the whites" as it is commonly called, a condition harbored in the vagina of a female, can also cause infection of the prostate.

A type of amoeba has been named in prostatic conditions. It was linked to the patient having drunk water which was polluted with this amoeba.

Even the foreskin of the penis has been blamed as a source of prostate infection. This authoritative author and medical man claims that in the super excellent climate created by the folded layers of the foreskin, along with the urinary drippings, germs are harbored and develop and can contaminate the prostate gland. However, when one realizes that Moslems and Jews who have their foreskin removed suffer as much from prostate troubles as do the un-circumcized, I am inclined to rule out the validity of this germ-prepuce theory.

Constipation

Chronic constipation is widely suggested as a contributor to prostate troubles. However, it must be clearly recognized that anyone who suffers from constipation is heir to a great many constitutional ailments and it might aggravate an existing prostate condition as well.

One has but to examine a chart showing the location of the prostate (See illustration facing Page 62) and its proximity to the rectum to quickly realize that a stuffed or loaded rectum could be a serious contributory factor in prostatic derangement.

However, inasmuch as it affects the prostate, I would like to point out what I believe to be a most important underlying consideration and that is that it is not so much the constipation in itself as the straining and the forcing and the pressure that is brought to bear in the region of the rectum in trying to obtain an evacuation. There is a strong likelihood that an improper evacuation or a rectum continually filled with foecal matter can cause disturbances and irritation to the prostate gland. But I am more inclined to believe that the forcing and straining is by far the more serious contributor to trouble with the prostate. I would strongly urge my readers to do everything possible to avoid this unnecessary, harmful and grievous practice. As a general rule, I do not suggest frequent enemas. On the other hand, there is no question about it that an enema is preferable to this violent over-exertion of bodily functions.

Remember, it is not vitally essential that you have a bowel movement at any given hour. It could be later, it could be earlier. So, therefore, it is not necessary to sit at the appointed hour and force yourself into a movement at any price.

MEDIAN SECTION OF THE MALE PELVIS

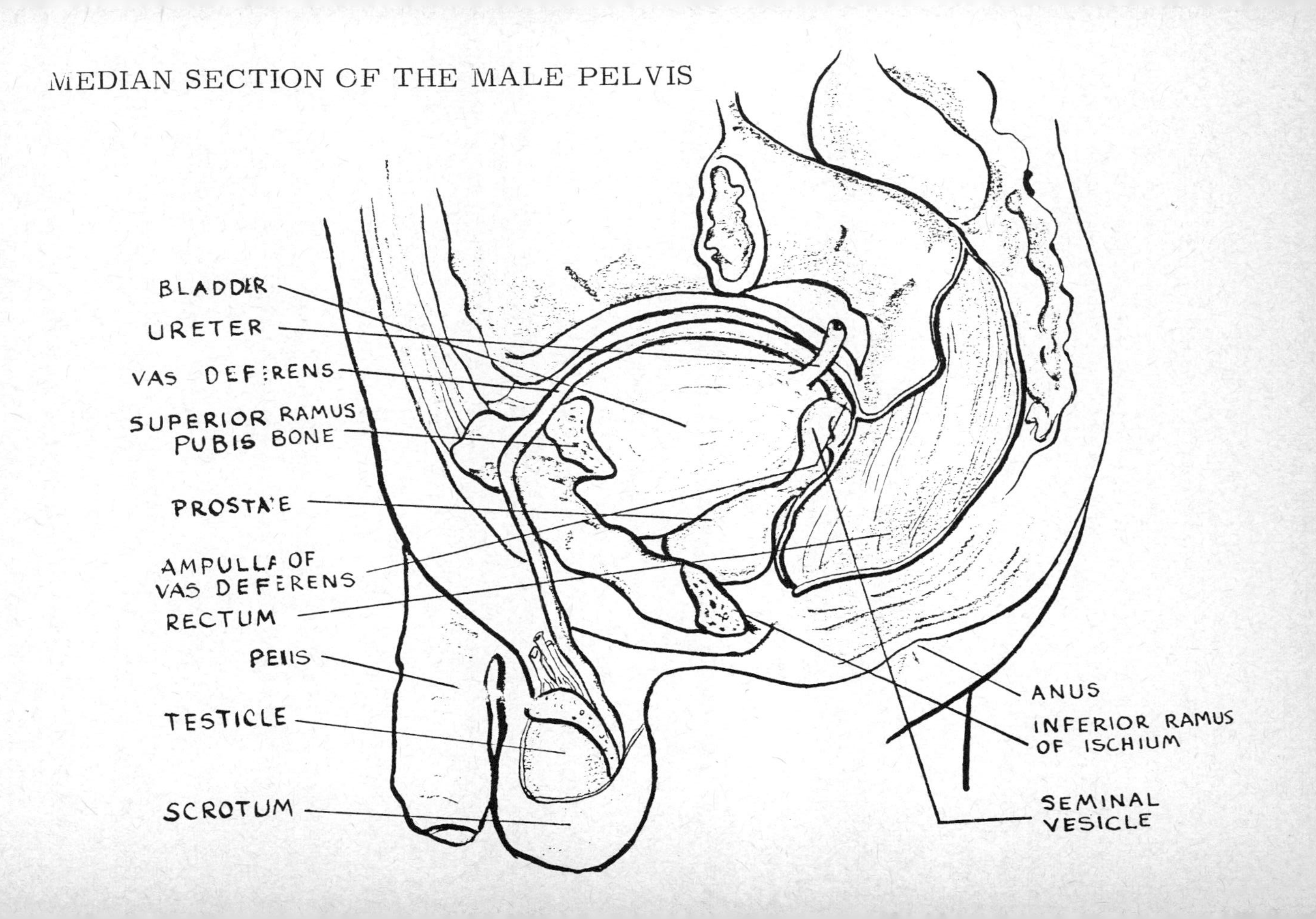

Salt

Frequent urination or polyuria, which is usually followed by or associated with frequent nocturnal urination, is found regularly in prostate disorders. It is my belief that this condition is frequently brought about by the continued excessive use of refined common or table salt.

Ragnar Berg shows through years of research that the body stores and builds up enormous supplies of sodium chloride. Evidently it builds up this store because it cannot quickly excrete it. That is, usually it can only excrete a certain amount per day and all that it cannot excrete it stores in various organs, glands, fat and tissue in the system and even in the blood. The body eliminates salt as quickly as it can and as rapidly as ample quantities of water are provided. The body doesn't care where or when or how it gets rid of it, as long as it does. Thus, if it can do so during your sleeping hours, you are awakened with the desire to urinate.

This may not at all indicate prostate trouble. What it really indicates is that your body is loaded with salt and of course its means of elimination -- water.

So one of the simplest and most direct remedies is right here and now to stop using salt of any kind of in any inorganic form. However, by merely stopping the use of salt today, we do not expect or believe that tomorrow you will be all right because that isn't true. According to the same author, Ragnar Berg, it will take not only months but often years to get rid of all the salt stored in the body. Furthermore, while you are still taking salt in your food or drink, you will never get rid of the salt that is stored in your body. It is only when you completely abstain from the use of inorganic salt that the body clearing process can take place ... and even from the day you start, it will take months or even years.

Therefore, you see, you cannot expect relief quickly. But if you abstain, the day will come when you will no longer have to get up nights to urinate ... and maybe your prostate condition will automatically clear itself up in this manner.

The excessive amount of salt in your body could be the chief reason that your body must resort to nocturnal urination. When you stop taking salt into your body, the day excretions of urine will normally suffice to rid your body of the salt. Then you will be able to sleep the night through without getting up to urinate.

Prior to 1923 Ragnar Berg said: "For more than 30 years we have known that the sodium ion has a paralyzing effect upon the activities both of the kidneys and of the ureters."

This quotation is also from Ragnar Berg's famous book "Vitamins": "In my own writings I have always insisted that the excretion of sodium chloride is a slow business, and that in persons who have been accustomed to consume an abundance of common salt, months or years of deprivation must elapse before the stores of sodium chloride in the body are depleted."

Then he goes on to include the chlorine ion in this category.

It is also a known fact that the salt does cause temporary paralysis of the sphincter muscles which lead from the bladder to the urethra.

Monosodium Glutamate

This is an extraordinarily emphatic warning concerning the use of monosodium glutamate, which is also known as ajinomoto, sodium glutamate, glutacyl, Chinese seasoning, MSG, Accent, Zest and Glutavene. There may also be other names with which I am not familiar.

It is the monosodium salt of the naturally occurring L-form of glutamic acid and it is produced by hydrolysis of vegetable proteins. Monosodium glutamate is 86.98% glutamic acid.

This produce is made from the wastes of beet sugar molasses by acid hydrolysis. Wheat gluten and corn gluten wastes are also used in its manufacture.

Throughout the Orient -- for example, in China and Japan -- they make their monosodium glutamate from the wastes of soya beans.

When you buy it at most food and department stores, it is generally in a white crystaline powder form.

Now the magic of monosodium glutamate lies in the fact that when used with salt, it imparts a decidedly rich meat-like taste to practically any food. Monosodium glutamate would be practically useless without the use of common salt or sodium chloride. Salt must be present to effect this rich taste.

The Chinese learned to use it many centuries ago because it imparted a strong meat-like flavor to vegetable and grain dishes, which in reality contained very little or no meat. In this manner they made a wee bit of meat go a long way.

A 1% concentration of MSG gives food a sweetish taste or flavor.

Monosodium glutamate is also used to improve the taste of tobacco.

Now here is what monosodium glutamate actually does to the body. It causes alkalosis and hypokalemia. Here is the clincher ... it increases fluid retention in the body.

I maintain that the continued use of food containing quantities of monosodium glutamate, Accent or Zest, or whatever else it might be called, will, as sure as fate, lead to trouble with your kidneys, your bladder, your urethra, and your prostate.

If you have had bouts of retention or excessive urination after eating Chinese dishes and foods, now you know the true reason. Therefore, a word to the wise is sufficient.

Wheat

This is a note concerning the cause of prostate disorders that I am rather reluctant to bring up. The reason I am most reluctant to make this knowledge public is because it will make our troubled lives even more difficult ... and I have no desire to make things more difficult than they already are.

The truth seems to be emerging,

according to my studies, that as long as we consume large quantities of wheat in various forms and wheat products in general we will continue to have troubles with our prostates. It seems that things like bread, cake, biscuits, spaghetti, macaroni, cookies, doughnuts and a hundred and one other things that are made with wheat have to go by the board or be used as food in much smaller quantities. I suggest that wheat products be replaced by other foods if we are to retain our health.

Of course wheat and wheat products have been attacked by various authorities and there appears to be ample justification for their position. Upon examination it seems to me that their stand is well founded. Let me now make my personal attitude clear. It is not wheat as wheat or wheat 'per se' to which I am objecting. It is wheat fragmented, processed, baked, boiled or cooked. Some major changes, chemical or otherwise, take place in wheat and turn it from a normal, beneficial grain to a harmful substance.

If you have doubts as to whether or not I am on the right trail, I beg of you to consider the nations that use little or no wheat -- countries like China, Burma, Thailand, Ethiopia, Borneo and others. Upon investigation you will find that prostatic disease is practically non-existent, whereas in the wheat-consuming countries, particularly the Western world, prostate disorders are rampant.

Now I am offering you no conclusive proof concerning the advantages of rice over wheat but the facts are worth investigating. Citing wheat and bakery products as a foremost causative factor is, I must admit, a theory ... and I am theorizing.

Consider Furfural

Some time ago it was brought to my attention that a product known as furfural, which is a bi-product in the milling of wheat, soy beans, and other grains, is used in various ways in the food industry. One of its uses, I understand, is in coffee or canned coffee because it enhances the pleasing coffee aroma.

A well known biochemist, in fact a very able one, informed me that he believes there is a direct link between this furfural and prostatic disorders. Therefore, remembering that furfural is a bi-product of the milling industry, specifically of wheat, this lends a bit of strength to my argument.

Lack of Natural Essential Oils

Now I would like to bring to light a theory concerning what I believe to be a major cause of prostate troubles. In fact, I humbly but sincerely suggest that it could be the cause or the most important cause of prostate troubles. This is an entirely new concept but a vital, intensively studied concept ... so listen!

I wish to make it crystal clear that I consider an important contributor to prostate disorders to be the fact that in this day and age few if any men ingest enough natural oils into their bodies to maintain their sexual organs in sound healthy condition. This of course also refers to the excretions of the sexual organs. Most of the oils that are taken into the human body are so highly refined or chemically treated or heated or plasticized or synthesized that the human body is unable to properly assimilate and utilize them. In fact, processed refined oils do not contain essential nutrients required by the body for normal functions, including sexual relations. Thus, the body is starved -- yes, I mean actually and literally starved -- for the nutrients that would normally be contained in these oils in their natural state and which would aid in the function of the sexual and other secretions. That is why many authorities in giving treatments for prostate disorders recommend the use of vitamin F and such items as pumpkin, sunflower and flax seed ... because when ingesting this type of food, one gets the oils in a natural, assimilable form.

It is obvious that the more a man indulges in sex, the more orgasms or ejaculations he will have. Each ejaculation costs a man something. I don't mean in dollars and cents or that he must pay a prostitute for the service. But it is costing something of himself. It is known that the seminal fluid is many times more potent than blood. Therefore, each time a man ejaculates he is giving something of his body and something of himself. It is also recognized that the semen is an oily substance. Remember, nature must continually replenish this supply of oily seminal fluid. There is no other way, this substance must be supplied to the body in the form of food.

First and foremost, allow me to inform you that there is no refined vegetable or animal oil on the market that nourishes the body and permits the body to fully and properly utilize it. Yes, I am referring to things like butter, milk, cream, oil, shortening and fats in any form. I contend that the body cannot properly metabolize this fat and that most of it is excreted in the faeces or stored in various organs, tissues and glands. All oils of vegetable origin are fragmented foods and in practically all cases they are chemically treated by means of a solvent which is used to extract the oil from the seeds. Then, because of the various processes through which the oil passes, as well as further chemical treatments, it is no longer a food but becomes a plastic or a strictly inorganic substance not any better and often worse than mineral oil.

Now you may argue that the oil as found in butter or in cream or in lard or suet would be satisfactory and that it would be organic and thus assimilable by the body. However, I contend that animal fats that have been pasteurized or heated to high temperatures are also in the same category as the inorganic or mineral oils and the body is unable to assimilate them. Yes, you may take any oil you like -- linseed oil, olive oil, safflower oil, sunflower oil, soya oil, cottonseed oil, walnut oil or apricot oil -- but they have all been either solvent-extracted or processed under extremely high temperatures or chemically treated. In any event, they are rendered such that the body is unable to utilize them. Therefore, as time goes on and man indulges in normal or excessive sexual relations, the stock, the source, the supply of oil becomes depleted ... and I contend that this is a major contribution to prostatic disorders.

To illustrate my point of view I will repeat a bit of conversation that I had with a friend who said, "Do you mean to tell me that the oils I get in my salads or with my French fries or with my fried foods are useless and non-nutritive?"

"Yes, I contend that that is absolutely true!"

"Would you also state," he questioned further, "that the butter I eat, the cream I have in my coffee and the fat that is found on my steaks are not assimilable by my body?"

My answer is that if the steak is eaten rare and the dairy products unpasteurized and most of the enzymes or microorganisms that are normally found in fat have not been destroyed, then your body would be able to derive some of the nutrients from it and metabolize them.

It is a fact that the body does get some fat from various things that we eat; for example, from nuts and seeds eaten without processing and that have not been permitted to become rancid, meats that have not been over-cooked and perhaps from butter or cream or milk that has not been pasteurized.

This trace of fat that the human body manages to extract from your diet keeps the body in some form of health and well-being. It further enables a man to perform the occasional sexual act.

It has been found that pumpkin seeds, for example, do help people who are suffering from disorders involving the genital organs. Why pumpkin seeds were accented I do not know except that in an experiment that was tried, pumpkin seeds were used. It is my belief, and I am quite certain that it is correct, that all edible seeds and nuts contain oils that can be utilized by the body.

I urge the use of seeds in the diet but they must be untreated seeds, they must be fresh seeds and they must not have their husks removed in advance. I suggest pumpkin seeds, squash seeds, sunflower seeds, sesame, flax and all kinds of nuts.

I have found that the best, the handiest and the most reasonably priced seeds of all are flax and sesame. But as they are rather difficult or not completely pleasant to eat as they are, I have suggested that they be mixed into a concoction with flax, sesame and honey in equal parts. Put the ingredients in a jar and stir them up and you have not only a pleasant tasting, appetizing, delicious food or candy but a nutritional food that is hard to beat. Not only do you get the oil that your body is sorely in need of but you get a comparatively well balanced, nutritional diet at the same time. There is no reason why other raw seeds and grains could not be used.

If you are using nuts for the same purpose, then I would strongly suggest that you buy nuts in the shell and crack them yourself so that none of the nutritional value will be lost and the nuts will not become rancid.

Nuts that have been shelled and kept under heat are worse than useless. In fact, I suggest that they may be harmful. Make sure that your nuts or seeds are fresh.

Phenacetin a Contributor?

Recently I came across a story concerning a drug known as phenacetin. This drug is widely used along with aspirin and other analgesics as a means of relieving headaches. It has been broadly stated by many authorities that this drug, phenacetin, does cause kidney damage and often death.

Here is a report I read recently, under the heading "Phenacetin Suspected as Source of Kidney Trouble":

"Some manufacturers of headache remedies containing phenacetin are still refusing to accept reports linking prolonged use of that drug with kidney damage and sometimes death. Two years ago when the danger was first detected, several drug firms dropped phenacetin from their formulas. The makers of Anacin were among those who abandoned it, continuing to make a product under the same name but containing only aspirin and caffeine. Other companies stuck with the headache pill ingredient, however, hoping to keep it available to headache-prone Americans who often feel that aspirin alone isn't strong enough to cure their pain. The fuss over phenacetin has refused to die down, however. Reports on side effects have continued to come in and the Food and Drug Administration recently required that a warning label citing possible kidney damage be placed on headache remedies containing the compound.

"One of the large drug companies has taken the position that evidence against the ingredient in its widely-sold product Empirin is 'circumstantial,' and 'no cause and effect relationship has been proven.' It has prepared a comprehensive review and bibliography of research questioning reports on the relationship between kidney disease and phenacetin. In a letter to a leading health publication, the president of the company said, 'So far we have not been able to find substantial or worthwhile evidence to convict the single drug -- phenacetin -- or, for that matter, to specifically point the finger of suspicion against it. We are hoping the studies on animals with induced pyelonephritis (kidney disease) and an epidemiologic study now under way will provide more information to clarify the clinical impressions that a number of physicians seem to have with respect to phenacetin.'

"Studies on rats and dogs have confirmed the company's contention that 'kidney lesions of the type observed in man and ascribed to the abuse of phenacetin-containing drugs were not seen in these animals,' he added. The company also lists six editorials appearing in leading medical journals which take the position that the real danger lies in the abuses of not only phenacetin but other analgesic compounds in the headache remedies.

"That argument was slapped down recently by a researcher at the Royal Children's Hospital in Melbourne, Australia, however. Dr. Paul Ross said, 'Of the various combinations used when renal disease has been associated with a high intake of analgesics, only phenacetin has been found to be the common factor.' He continued, 'Although the evidence linking chronic phenacetin intake and renal disease is not conclusive since this association has not been proven experimentally, it is strongly suggested and has been repeatedly confirmed clinically.'

"Other researchers have also spoken out against indiscriminate use of phenacetin-containing preparations. Just recently the Pharmaceutical Society of Great Britain warned, 'So insidious are its ill effects on the kidneys that the risk of prolonged use has only recently been discovered and people taking it do not connect its use with such illness.' Commenting on the Society's warning, Drug and Therapeutics Bulletin urged British physicians to 'accept that there is a risk rather than to belittle it.' It has been recently reported that a prominent group of American doctors representing the Medical Letter advised that over-the-counter preparations containing the drug should not be recommended even for limited use by patients who can tolerate aspirin. Perhaps the most damaging report is a recent British Medical Journal editorial. It concluded, 'At present it would seem wise not to prescribe analgesic drug mixtures containing phenacetin as a long-term measure to any patient, or at all to patients with diabetes or disease of the renal tract'."

I would like to warn against the use of drugs, more specifically any drug or preparation containing phenacetin. If phenacetin causes renal or kidney troubles, then I am afraid it will also do harm to the prostate. Remember, it must pass through the kidneys into the ureters and down into the prostate and through the urethra before it can be voided in the urine. Therefore, I contend that it can and does cause prostate complications. So I would remind you most emphatically to avoid any drugs, especially those containing phenacetin.

Water Softeners

Just what part water softeners play in prostate disorders I admit that I am unable to say but because of the very serious effects and changes in the constituents of the water which are brought about by chemicals used in the softeners, I would emphatically warn that water softeners could be a serious factor in health and disease. I have no specific charges to make against water softeners at this writing but I do wish to point out that they effect profound, definite chemical changes in the water and for anyone who is suffering from prostate trouble I would urge against using water that has been softened or treated in any way. I would further advise against the use of water softeners of any kind or description where the water is to be used for drinking or cooking.

Cooked Root Vegetables

Just a while ago I came across a statement to the effect that people who have a high consumption rate of root vegetables like potatoes, sweet potatoes, carrots and parsnips, and who eat them cooked in various ways, also suffer from prostatic troubles. The indication was that these cooked root vegetables created some disturbance which affected the prostate. I would suggest that the chemical changes that took place in the cooking are suspect rather than the vegetables as mentioned.

High Protein Diet

It is suggested that a heavy protein diet causes malfunctions or diseases of the kidneys. By and large, the literature that I have pored over and digested has clearly indicated that a heavy protein diet is a forceful influence in prostatic disease. Please bear in mind that a heavy protein diet does not necessarily mean meat or fish. Grains, nuts, cheese, eggs and many other foods are also well known as being primarily protein. I would further suggest that a high protein diet may be a contributor to enlarged prostate and I would advise anyone who has any sign of trouble with his prostate to definitely avoid a high protein diet.

It is also suggested that high protein diet is a virile diet but there is no sound, logical or scientific basis for this belief or assumption.

Petting Without Sexual Gratification

I wonder just how big a part consistent petting without sexual gratification plays in prostatic disorders. I think it is recognized that petting without gratification is too widely practised in our modern society -- especially in our youth. Now I am not advocating that this practice be stopped, nor am I suggesting that it be permitted that the couple involved be allowed to partake of sexual relationship to avoid the harm of the persistent petting. I am only bringing this to the attention of my readers for what it might be worth.

It would appear as though being aroused to a high pitch of sexual desire and then being frustrated by denial might have a harmful effect upon the prostate gland, if not upon the whole nervous system of the male human being. I place this right alongside masturbation as being an important contributing factor.

Going even further, it is a fact that among all other animals on earth every female is a sexual object or target and it is just a matter of being in the right place at the right time during the mating season and copulation takes place. With man it is entirely different. No doubt most men would like to do this too but unfortunately, because of restraints, rules and regulations, customs and conventions, he finds himself with his desires and passions going up and down like a see-saw, perhaps many times a day. One must admit that these drastic surges would be a pre-disposing factor in prostatic disease. I'm sure that a normal, vigorous, youthful male human being, whether he is going to school or working, finds himself sexually aroused and dumped into cold water probably a dozen or more times a day. This is definitely not a healthy practice or way of life. It strikes me as a strong pre-disposing force.

Possible Primary Cause

My conclusion concerning the positive causative factors of prostate troubles is in a state of flux. This I admit without any reservations, though I feel I have studied all factors pertaining to the prostate as no other man living or dead has done.

It is my belief that your prostate troubles began the first time your dear old mother slapped your bottom when you wet your diaper or your pants. No, 'tis not the slap but the implication that you cannot, in accordance with the rules of civilization, urinate where and when you would.

I do sincerely believe I could lay down a set of rules that would prevent this condition from developing but this pattern would have to be started in babyhood and it would mean giving up many pleasures that we have learned to accept as a part of our way of life. More about this in another chapter.

Section B -- Pinpointing the Factors

My search for data on the prostate has been going on now for many years and I believe I am acquainted with what are generally accepted and conceded to be causative factors in prostate difficulties. I'll list the causative factors in what I believe to be the order of their importance:

1. Not heeding nature's call as demanded.
2. Thwarting the sexual climax -- coitus interruptus.

3. Lack of natural oils in the diet.
4. Chemical additives in food.
5. Sedentary occupations.
6. Salt in food.
7. Coffee, tea and other beverages.
8. Hot seasonings and condiments in food.
9. Masturbation.
10. Venereal diseases.
11. Sexual over-indulgence or forcing the climax.
12. Drugs and their side effects.
13. Coitus prolongatus.
14. Too much fluid in the system when retiring.
15. Coitus reservatus.
16. Straining at stool.
17. Insufficient sexual relations.
18. Incorrect posture and bad sitting habits -- prolonged periods in distorted, unnatural positions.
19. Long periods of automobile riding without exercise.
20. High protein diet.
21. The use of alcoholic beverages.

There are no doubt many other contributing factors but I have only been able to track down the ones listed above as having a definite relationship with prostatic disorders.

While most of the factors outlined above are widely known and accepted, there are a few that no other author, in writing about the prostate, has ever given. I believe I have delved deeply into the situation and am presenting facts, clinical proof and observations not generally brought out into the open.

Perhaps you, like some authorities, look askance at or prefer to ignore the theory that insufficient sex can be a contributing factor. In passing, I would like to relate two specific instances I have come across which bear out this theory. The reason I want to bring these case histories before you is because seldom if ever is this factor mentioned in available literature as being an important causative factor.

Case No. 1:

Bob Forbes was a school teacher. His wife was an extremely busy woman. Between her social activities and her home she had very little time for anything else.

Bob began to have urination difficulties as well as accompanying pains in the groin. After this condition had persisted for some time and was growing worse he went to see a physician. After careful examination and study his physician sent him to a specialist. After a routine examination and discussion the specialist asked him how often he indulged in sexual intercourse. He told the physician that he had intercourse about once a month and sometimes even less frequently.

"But don't you have the desire for more frequent intercourse?" the specialist asked him.

"Yes, I could stand more and often feel that I need sex more frequently."

"Then why don't you indulge in it more often?"

Bob, somewhat embarrassed, told the specialist, "My wife is so busy and when I do get around to it she is usually so tired and indisposed that we just don't indulge."

The specialist said, "From my examination I would say that your condition is caused by insufficient use of your prostate gland. I would suggest that you talk to your wife and explain that the situation will become much more aggravated unless you indulge in more frequent intercourse."

Forbes went home and laid the matter before his wife and, being an understanding woman and loving her husband and wanting to keep him alive and healthy, she agreed to have more frequent sexual relations.

From then on Mr. Forbes' prostatic troubles gradually cleared up and finally disappeared. He is some years older now without even the faintest sign of prostate trouble.

Case No. 2:

This was related to me by a good friend in New York. His son had difficulties with his prostate in his late teens. Yes, this is absolutely true and can be verified. This difficulty continued until his middle 20's, when he consulted a doctor. The physician made the usual examination and he was quite shocked when, upon questioning him, he found that this young man had never indulged in sexual relations. I presume my readers will recognize this as a most unusual situation because I doubt if one boy or man in 1000 reaches the age of 25 without ever having indulged in sex. Now I did not question my friend so I do not know whether or not his son practised masturbation.

The physician suggested marriage. This advice was followed within a few months ... the lad took himself a wife and from that time onward he had no further trouble with his prostate.

Section C -- Civilization's Contribution

What part does civilization play in prostate disease? This is a burning question and one that few authorities would attempt to answer. I consider it a vitally important factor but it has seldom if ever been mentioned by other investigators and authors.

The fact that the older medical literature fails to specifically mention prostate diseases indicates that prostate diseases were either uncommon or unknown. I gravely doubt that there was such a thing as positive prostate derangement over 100 years ago. But it is reasonable to assume that because of advancements in diagnosis and improved technological methods during the past century, conditions that were once thought to be of kidney, bladder or urinary origin are now accepted as being caused by an impaired prostate.

My quest at the moment is to establish whether or not our modern way of living is to blame for prostate diseases. I do not seek to blame civilization nor am I begging the question. The fact, however, is clear that young men today have prostate trouble and this was not true 50 or 100 years ago.

Just let us go back 100 years. That isn't too far back by dimensions or measurements of history. I think I'd be safe in saying that a hundred years ago 99 people out of 100 performed some form of manual labor. Even if you were a shop-keeper you would still have had a fair amount of manual labor to do in the course of a day. The only people not called upon to perform any physical labor would have been the wealthy, the healers, the bankers, the bookkeepers and the clerks ... but I dare say in those days not one person in 100 would have fit into these categories.

The further back you go in history the fewer were the number of people who were not called upon to do physical labor in performance of their occupations and daily living.

Let's examine the situation today. In my organization that involves approximately 10 employees only one man does any serious physical labor. Some do a bit of physical work, like assembling orders and wrapping parcels, but I want to rcpeat, approximately one man out of 10 does actual heavy physical work.

Now you may say that men in factories all do physical labor, but I will beg to disagree. They have machines to do most of the heavy work. All a man does is feed these machines, using but a few muscles of the many in his body. Nevertheless, I am not going to go any deeper into the breakdown of the number of people who do physical work but you can easily gather what I am driving at ... that the loss of physical activity can be, and I believe is, a most comprehensive factor in the increase in prostatic disorders.

I realize that in America there are thousands of men, such as truck drivers and stevedores, as well as laborers in construction and other allied industries, who do a fair amount of physical labor but they represent but a small part of the total population. And I am willing to wager that the incidence of prostate disorders among them reaches a low, low -- probably the lowest in our society.

Upon careful thought, all the men that I know who have had prostate trouble (and there are many) are executives, clerks, salesmen and other sedentary workers.

I contend that in our present economy only one person in ten performs actual physical work. It is my firm contention and belief that nature intended man to perform physical work, to earn his daily bread by the sweat of his face, and not sit on his fanny and permit it to spread and grow fatter. I suggest that therein lies one of the basic reasons for the great increase in prostatic troubles. A healthy prostate can only be found in an active, healthy male. Therefore, I suggest the sedentary occupations of modern man as an important suspect in the cause of prostate trouble. One way to avoid this trouble is to exercise as much as possible ... and walking in itself is not enough.

While preparing this manuscript I read a most interesting book about a tribe of aborigines in the deserts of Australia who have never known the hand of civilization. The author of this book tells of finding some of these strange people. He describes how they urinated or defecated at the instant nature called. He even tells about one case where a man was eating and urinating at the same time.

Here I quote from the book:

"He sat back on his heels and urinated in the sand, involuntarily it seemed, without apparently knowing or caring that he was doing so."

Then again later on in the book:

"As he squatted before me, urinating again in the sand while continuing to eat, I felt that he was by far the most primitive man we had seen."

Please don't confuse the situation and think that I am advocating such procedure or a return to stone age practices. What I am trying to say is that this aborigine was in the process of eating when he had a call by nature and as a true child of nature, he responded to that call there and then. With him there were no other considerations or any of civilization's demands or rules or regulations to be concerned about. It is probably that nature intended that when the urine had to be emitted all else must go by the board and the urine must flow. The same probably holds true for defecation, or even sex relations.

Withholding urine so as to urinate at a fixed time or place is definitely not a part of normal animal behaviour. Therefore, because civilization makes this demand upon man and it is adhered to to varying and even fantastic exceptional degrees, I suggest that withholding or controlling the flow of urine *is* the foremost cause of prostate disorders.

From my on-the-spot investigations I have found that farmers suffer less prostate trouble than any other segment of our civilized population and I guess the reason for this is clear. A farmer, when he is working about his farm, can avail himself of instantaneous emptying of the bladder whenever the need arises because he spends a great deal of his time out in his fields or in the stables. The facts speak for themselves. I repeat, farmers have the lowest incidence of prostate trouble of any segment of our population.

I would point out that a human being is the only creature on the face of the earth who is apt to indulge in sexual relations 365 days of the year. All other animals indulge in sex in a predetermined cycle -- in the rutting or mating season only.

Further, man is the only animal who indulges in sex for other purposes than procreation. Man is the only animal who drinks alcoholic beverages and he is the only one who smokes. Man is also the only animal who drinks tea and coffee. Man is the only living thing who cooks his food, too.

Because prostatic conditions are unknown among any other animals in their native habitat, these factors bear emphasis. I must here concede that dogs are also known to have prostate trouble. But remember, dogs are domesticated and they must, of course, control their urine, as taught and demanded by their masters, and they are invariably fed civilized, chemicalized and refined foods.

Somehow cats seem to handle the situation in a more practical light. For example, if a cat wishes out, it will sit itself near a door or passageway before the need becomes urgent and the moment the door is opened by someone going out or coming in, it is the first to exit. Besides, a cat will avail itself of an open window if it desires 'out' or use the cellar or a coal bin, a pile of ashes or debris. In fact, a cat is much more realistic and adaptable to such things than either a human being or a dog and therefore, the retention angle seldom confronts it.

Now you will quickly recognize that most domesticated dogs do not have the opportunity to indulge in regular sex relations at will because they are controlled within the confines of the average home or held under a leash or perhaps a bitch isn't available. On the other hand, tom-cats, for example, do get out and do have sexual relations or mating sprees as is evidenced by the meowing and the screeching that takes place at night. And according to my veterinarian informants, cats do not have prostate troubles.

There appears to be little if any doubt that prostate trouble of various kinds is one of the diseases of civilization, for when one studies the incidence of prostate disorders in the different countries throughout the world the figures clearly indicate that the Caucasian race is affected with more prostate troubles than any other race.

It would be a safe bet to say that the Caucasians suffer more prostate trouble than all of the other races combined. So apart from being a disease of civilization, it is essentially a disorder common to the White race. This definitely is not intended to suggest that the Yellow and Black races are uncivilized but a suggestion that their social customs are different. Orientals and the Black race seem to be generally immune to prostatic disorders. However, I am not speaking of Orientals or Blacks who live among the White peoples and have followed the white man's ways.

Actual studies and surveys made in Africa, Japan, Indonesia and China clearly show that in these countries there are comparatively few cases of prostate troubles and tumors.

There are a great many opinions on this subject. One argument given to repudiate this statement hinges on the claim that among the Orientals or the Blacks, medical treatment and hospitals are comparatively rare and, therefore, the incidence of prostatic difficulties would not be discovered. Mind you, I think that this argument has some logic behind it but, nevertheless, a condition as serious and as common as prostate trouble is in the West would most certainly come to the surface if it prevailed in the Orient or in Africa.

In my travels through various countries throughout the world I found that in some of the remote spots the people live just as they lived 100 years ago ... yes, and in some of the more remote places, hundreds of years ago. Please don't doubt me because I speak the truth and can prove it to anyone who is willing to question me and listen or go to these remote places in person.

In those areas I doubt if the incidence of prostate trouble has increased. I contend that there is something in our newly found, improved, mechanized, synthetic way of life that is contributing in a marked manner to the high incidence of prostate disorders. It might be our beverages, it might be the food we eat, it might be the air we breathe. It could be the contributions of the motor age and soft living. Then again, it might be due to the changeover from physical to sedentary occupations.

One doctor who had spent most of his practising life in Burma told me that the chief reason few native Burmese had prostate trouble was because they didn't live long enough. He claimed they seldom live beyond 50 and as prostate conditions usually afflict older people, therefore, they died before the prostate caused much trouble. This is one doctor's view but I do not regard it as valid.

It is granted that no one knows precisely how much prostatic disease does exist in those lands. There is, however, a most important point to take into consideration here. In talking to physicians and surgeons who have worked in the Orient and Africa, I have invariably been informed that prostate troubles are seldom found and are almost unknown in these areas. Even here in America it is a definite, accepted fact that the colored people and the Chinese suffer less from prostate trouble than do the whites. You can check with any doctor who has had experience in such cases for confirmation of this statement.

But even if the Orientals and the colored folk living in America had as high an incidence of prostate troubles as the whites it would cause me no great surprise because after all, if they live here among us, they would eventually live much as we do and therefore would be affected more or less by similar diseases.

In my open discussions with laymen, physicians and sociologists concerning prostate disorders one of them came up with a rather interesting angle. He said, "Is it not true that among the white races, especially in the West, there are more taboos, restrictions, complications and difficulties regarding sexual relations than are found anywhere else in the world?"

This question was presented to me some time ago and I begged off for time to study and consider that matter at my leisure. After a great deal of reflection I had to admit that here in America we do have more taboos and rules and regulations against sex than are found in most other countries in the world. Now I will grant that this could be a most important factor or a strong contributor to prostate diseases because the prostate gland is so interwoven with the sex organs and so readily affected by them that any complications regarding sex could have an adverse effect on the prostate and its connecting organs.

It is true, and no one can deny it, that the modern American male is concerned and surrounded with problems about sex from his early youth until his sexual organs no longer function. So if you consider the fears, the wonders, the infringements and the intricacies of the situation that develop and entwine with and around a man's sexual life, it is certainly something worthy of consideration when we ponder the causes of prostate disorders.

It is widely recognized that heart disease, cancer, arthritis and diabetes are definitely diseases of civilization. But there is no doubt about it, we must now add prostate diseases to this imposing list.

Then we must ask ourselves if chlorinated water is a factor in prostate disease? Or is chlorinated water a factor in any disease? It must be recognized that water is not the same once it has been treated with chlorine. However, as we are dealing here specifically with the prostate, that is where we will leave it.

Because prostate disease is proven to be a disease of higher or modern civilization, chlorination of our water supply as a causative factor must be taken into consideration. Chlorination of water supplies is followed only among the modern civilized peoples.

Chapter Seven

FOOD ADDITIVES AND THE PROSTATE

I have been unable to find any statistics showing an increase or decrease in the number of cases involving enlargement or degeneration of the prostate gland. While it is easy to get figures concerning cancer, heart disease, muscular dystrophy, diabetes and many other diseases, figures that would indicate whether or not prostatic disorders are on the increase are difficult if not impossible to find.

However, I don't think anyone will question my statement that prostatic conditions are definitely on the increase. Of course there are those who will claim that because medical science has increased the life span of man and because he is now living longer, prostatic conditions show up and therefore appear to be on the increase. The same argument is given for cancer and heart disease as well. In turn, I would challenge that medical science alone has given us an increase in life expectancy ... but we will not indulge in the pleasure of that argument at this time. So I will revert to my first statement, which I doubt if anyone can contradict, and that is that diseases or troubles involving the prostate are definitely increasing.

Now if I were to boldly and emphatically state that the use of chemicals in food has also increased greatly in the past 50 years, I doubt if anyone would challenge that statement either. So now I simply put two and two together and say that the use of chemicals has increased greatly and so have diseases of the prostate, and therefore the use of chemicals in food is the cause of prostatic conditions. Therefore, by all laws of simple logic. the case has been tried, proven and the culprit (chemicals in food) found guilty.

However, the use of aspirin has also increased greatly in the past 50 years ... and so has the use of oranges and other fruits, alcohol, coffee, tea and the different kinds of soft drinks. Then one might state that all of these things may be factors in prostatic conditions. But with this kind of reasoning, I must admit, we will get nowhere fast.

Data is not readily available to pinpoint exactly when chemicals began to be used in foods. However, for ages mankind has been using various types and kinds of preservatives which would prolong the keeping qualities of many foods.

The closest I can come to any conclusion regarding the advent of chemical treatments of foods is somewhere around 1850 when Liebig, the father of organic chemistry and probably the founding father of chemical preservatives in food, began to experiment with the chemical treatment of food.

Nevertheless, at the turn of the century chemical food additives seemed to be definitely on the increase as is clearly indicated by the fight that Dr. Harvey Wiley, the first boss of the Food and Drug, put up in the United States ... which is vividly told in his book, "A Crime Against the Food Laws."

Bread, of course, has been adulterated since time immemorial but all adulterations are not necessarily chemicals and thus, they are not always harmful.

However, broadly speaking, chemical additives did not become a factor in food until some time after the end of World War I, somewhere around 1920. Chemicals in foods became vitally important and were used in practically all processed foods by the time of the second World War ... and even more so by the time of the Korean War. Sustaining an army so far away on these chemically processed foods that did not spoil really brought food chemicals into the limelight.

For the first time "Big Business" began to be interested in food. You see, the chemical preservatives had eliminated many of the risks of spoilage caused by bacterial action. The Korean War proved the effectiveness and efficiency of food chemicals, and the modern machinery and new methods of processing completed the picture. Thus, it became possible to make shipments of enormous quantities of food across wide expanses and over long periods of time and permitted these foods to reach their destination without any bacterial deterioration and in what, to the naked eye, appeared to be perfect condition.

It was at this time that food chemicals came into their own. Since then the great leap forward has taken place until now you can buy no packaged, processed, canned or preserved food that does not contain anywhere from one to twenty, or even more, different chemical additives.

I don't know whether or not you accept the following statement but it is an absolute fact. No additive was ever put into a food to improve it ... that is from a nutritional point of view. Chemical additives are put into foods for many reasons, but never to improve the nutritional value.

In this volume I am dealing specifically with the prostate and therefore the reason why chemicals are put into foods is irrelevant ... but the fact remains that the use of chemicals in food is widespread and increasing by leaps and bounds. In fact, practically every processed, packaged food on the shelves of the supermarkets throughout America contains one or many chemical additives.

I would like at this point to deal with those chemical additives that are most frequently used in the greatest number of foods. Then I would also look into the chemicals added to the foods that are most widely used. I doubt if there is a handful of people in a thousand in America who do not use baked goods. Therefore, we will in due course deal with the chemicals contained in baked goods. I doubt if there is one person in a thousand who does not use refined salt in his food and so we will deal with the chemicals added to salt.

I doubt if there is one person in a hundred who does not use factory-processed jams, jellies, pickles or other canned fruit or vegetables. So we will also deal with the chemicals contained in these. Too, I will deal with the chemicals that are put into beer and soft drinks and into candy and ice cream and hot dogs and hamburgs. No one can deny that hamburgs are one of the most popular foods in North America.

It is my belief that after we have covered the most widely used foods and the chemicals that are added to them, we should have some form of a case that might indicate a contributing factor in prostate disorders.

So that my claims may be accepted, believed and substantiated I will, in every case, quote the source from which my data has been derived. I want it clearly understood that I am not building a case against anyone or any commodity. I am just relating the truth, the facts and the data as I found them. Furthermore, I would like to stress that I do not claim that chemicals in foods are the cause of all prostate difficulties. I do, however, sincerely believe that they are a suspect and can be a contributory factor. Just how big a part food chemicals play in the matter I do not know but I present the information for you to read and study ... and you can reach your own conclusions.

Speaking strictly for myself, I gave up the use of any food that contains a chemical additive more than three years ago. It is possible that some of the foods that I eat contain some chemical additives of which I am not aware but I dare say that 99% of all the foods I eat are free of any chemical additives whatsoever.

I will, in the following pages, give the various chemicals that are put into such daily, vital, accepted foods as white and whole wheat flour, bread, cakes, leavening agents, salt, beverages, meats, pickles, jams, jellies, cheese, oils, fruit juices, salad dressings, ice cream, margarine, synthetic sweeteners and coffee.

It is not my intention in this volume to go into any great detail concerning chemicals in food or the harm they do or the good they do. I am only interested here in chemicals in food that may contribute to or cause problems or harm to the prostate gland. So I will deal with such things that I have found contribute in some way or manner to the disorders of the genital and excretory organs.

From my studies it would appear that the harm lies in foods that form the major part of our diet and not so much in the foods that we eat only occasionally or as treats or titbits. Let us, for example, deal with the chemicals used in cakes, bread and meats and other food items used every day. I am not dealing with the chemicals used in sprays or insecticides on vegetables and fruits because many of these are washed off or removed and tolerance levels have been set for them by various Government agencies. We will deal here only with the chemicals in foods as authorized by the Food and Drug Administration.

I'd like to point out that in some instances the labels on the processed foods give a warning or list the contents which will show the added chemicals. On the other hand, the law does not demand that all of the chemicals in foods be put on the label. For instance, on bread, on cake, soft drinks, ice cream, salt, meats, cheese and many others no warning or list of chemical additives is required.

Dr. Frank Bicknell, world renowned scientist, states: "Congenital abnormalities, physical and mental, are mainly caused by the alien substances added to food."

It is suggested that sodium bicarbonate can be a causative factor in kidney, bladder, urinary and prostatic conditions. As sodium bicarbonate is widely used in baking powders, this would be the same causative factor that is found in baked goods.

The following human toxicity is mentioned in the Merck Index, P. 946: "Average doses any route in presence of renal insufficiency or large doses any route in patients with normal renal function may cause alkalosis, irritability, restlessness, neuro-muscular hyperexcitability and tetany."

Here are the chemicals that are found in baking powder: Sodium bicarbonate, tartaric acid, potassium acid tartrate, monocalcium phosphate, sodium aluminum sulphate, sodium acid pyrophosphate.

Here are the chemicals that are added to salt: Magnesium carbonate, sodium thiosulphate, potassium iodide, tricalcium phosphate, aluminum silicate, hydrated calcium silicate, sodium aluminum silicate.

Here are some of the chemicals that are added to various meats: Sodium nitrite, sodium nitrate, potassium nitrate, potassium nitrite, sodium ascorbate and ascorbic acid.

Here are chemicals that are added to oils: Propyl gallate, benzoic acid, sulphurus acid, butylated hydroxyanisole, butylated hydroxytoluene, propylene glyco-nordhydroguiretic acid, propyonic acid, citric acid, sodium di-acetate.

Here are the chemicals added to flour: Oxides of nitrogen, chlorine, chlorine dioxide, nitrosyl chloride, benzoyl peroxide, calcium carbonate, calcium sulphate, dicalcium phosphate, magnesium carbonate, potassium aluminum sulphate, sodium aluminum sulphate, tricalcium phosphate, potassium bromate, ammonium persulphate, ammonium chloride.

Here are the chemicals that may be added to bread: Monoglycerides, diglycerides, ammonium chloride, calcium carbonate, calcium lactate, calcium sulphate, diammonium phosphate, dicalcium phosphate, monoammonium phosphate, potassium iodide, monocalcium phosphate, potassium bromate, potassium iodate, calcium peroxide, ammonium persulphate, potassium persulphate, propionic acid, sodium diacetate, sorbic acid and may include charcoals, carbon blacks, iron oxide, titanium dioxide, coal tar colors, aluminum or calcium lakes, arsenic, lead.

Cheese: Food color, pH adjusting agent, preservatives, calcium chloride.

Salad dressing: Sweetening agent, emulsifying agent, citric acid, tartaric acid, lactic acid, sequestering agent.

Evaporated milk: Added vitamin C, added vitamin D, disodium phosphate, sodium citrate.

Ice cream: Lactose, dextrose, glucose, flavoring preparation, cocoa or chocolate syrup, food coloring, pH adjusting agent, stabilizing agent, sequestering agent.

Shortening: Hydrogenated oil, preservative, antifoaming agent, stearyl monoglyceridyl citrate, monoglycerides, diglycerides, lactylated monoglycerides.

Cacao products: Hydroxides, carbonates, bicarbonates of sodium, potassium, magnesium.

It is not my intention to prove or claim that all of these chemicals affect or do harm to the prostate gland or the genito-urinal organs. However, investigations have clearly indicated that many of them do seriously affect the functions of the kidneys as well as the genital organs.

Furthermore, I would go on record as stating that if you want to take a decisive step towards preventing prostatic disorders, you should eat no food that contains a chemical additive ... and in this one way alone you may avoid malfunctions of the prostate, the kidneys and the bladder.

I'd also like to sound a warning against the use of chemical, synthetic or drug diuretics. Practically all of the known diuretics which cause or create a heavy flow of urine invariably eliminate not only the water or the urine from the system but deplete the body of various other vital elements. Therefore, any unnatural stimulation to urinate can cause various other disorders.

However, it is unlikely that the drinking of most natural herb teas -- for example, parsley -- would do more than eliminate the urine or water. I am not advising the use of parsley or other herbal diuretics but I am suggesting that the synthetic drug treatments for this purpose be avoided, for they invariably create more complications than they eliminate. They usually do more harm than good.

Chapter Eight

MEAT EATING AND ITS EFFECTS UPON THE PROSTATE

I have a specific purpose in connecting the eating of meat to prostate difficulties ... and it will reveal itself before the end of this chapter.

Further, I want it clearly understood, without any chance of error, that I am not a vegetarian nor am I opposed to the eating of meat.

It is my conviction that in the present day meat eating is a definite contributor to prostatic hypertrophy and I will offer what I deem to be proof ... clear, emphatic, undeniable proof of this statement. So read on with care and deliberation.

Diethylstilbestrol is what is known as a synthetic estrogen. Originally it was similar to the female sex hormone or estrogen which is found in the urine of pregnant mares as well as in the urine of stallions. Today it is simply a synthetic chemical which is added to the feed of fowl, beef cattle, sheep and sometimes hogs to quickly and unnaturally fatten or increase the weight of the animals.

Because this allegation against meat eating is a serious one, affecting a food eaten by 99% of the people of America, I want to explain that meat in itself is not my target or the guilty commodity. But I must mention that a heavy meat diet was suspect in kidney ailments long before diethylstilbestrol was ever added to our meat. No, in this instance I am not alluding to meat in any specific form. I clearly and without mincing matters mean meat as it is available today, treated with diethylstilbestrol, in any and all forms as purchased from any normal merchandising outlet.

Please follow me carefully in the following statement. At least 90% of all the meat sold in North America comes from animals that have been fed or are treated with diethylstilbestrol. It has been added to the feed of animals -- cattle, sheep and poultry -- for many years. The supposed purpose is to fatten the animals quickly, thus making them available for market in less time than normal. The reason, let me say, is not to improve the nutritional quality of the meat or to enhance its flavor but simply and truthfully to make it more profitable for the farmers, and of course, to enrich the chemical corporations that make and promote diethylstilbestrol.

Some years ago the government agencies in Canada and the United States banned the use of this drug which was then used as an implant in the form of a pellet behind the ear of cattle and in the neck of chickens. After some scandal the government regulation made operative at that time specified that it could not be used as an implant ... so now they use it in the feed.

The action of this drug is to create a disease within the body of the animal, causing it to swell like a goiter ... only this drug, diethylstilbestrol, causes the whole body to swell. And this diseased carcass passes the United States and Canadian government inspectors as first class or prime beef or poultry! But it is a fact that animals treated with this drug reach marketable weight sooner by some weeks than normal animals fed normal food without the drug.

For the sake of brevity we will use the abbreviated form of diethylstilbestrol, "stilbestrol."

While in Canada the use of stilbestrol for fattening chickens has been forbidden as an implant, I maintain that it is widely used in feeding and that practically all of the chickens on the market in Canada are treated with this drug. The carcasses of the chickens as well as the carcasses of cattle are loaded with stilbestrol. While the government makes a feeble pretense of trying to protect the public by a regulation that instructs the farmers not to feed stilbestrol within so many hours of the time they are slaughtered, this is just simple sleight of hand that has no value even if it were followed ... which in most cases it is not.

The simple, definite fact is that practically all of the meat you eat contains varying doses of stilbestrol. It is found in the entrails, it is found in the organs, it is found in the flesh and in the bones. Every part of the animal is loaded with stilbestrol. Cooking does not remove it. In fact, I suspect that it even concentrates it.

Now that I have established clearly and positively without any shadow of doubt that you do get your share of this drug with all of the meat you eat, let me point out to you that it is a definitely harmful drug that does cause not only prostatic hypertrophy but cancer as well. I will quote here from what is the most reliable and accepted authority in its field -- the Merck Index. I quote from Page 355 of the 1960 edition which is the latest edition as this book goes to press:

"DIETHYLSTILBESTROL

"Human Toxicity: Large doses may cause anorexia, nausea, vomiting, abdominal pain, diarrhea, headache, dizziness, lethargy, paresthesia, skin eruptions, breast engorgement, uterine bleeding, amenorrhea, loss of libido in males, dysuria, edema, congestive heart failure, mammary carcinoma in males. May cause or contribute to mammary or genital carcinoma in females. Caution: Hepatic disease. Benign prostatic hypertrophy. History of mammary or genital carcinoma or familial history of these. Should not be employed for uterine bleeding unless possibility of carcinoma has been thoroughly investigated.

"Vet. Use: Replacement therapy for underdeveloped females; incontinence, vaginitis of spayed bitches. To induce heat in anestrus. In uterine inertia pyometra. To check milk secretion pseudopregnancy; prevent conception in mismated bitches. In hypertrophy of prostate in dogs. Chemical caponization of poultry."

You will note that I have underlined "Benign prostatic hypertrophy" and also I have underlined that in veterinary use it is used "In hypertrophy of prostate in dogs." So there we have it. This selfsame drug that causes prostate hypertrophy is also used to treat the same disease. Just what kind of magic this is I am unable to say. I am only laying the facts before you. It is up to you to reach your own conclusion ... if you can!

From a scientific source in Great Britain it is claimed that diethylstilbestrol causes diminution in the size of the testes and penis, as well as loss of erections.

Vegetarians and natural hygienists frequently contend in their literature that people who eat flesh foods and animal products along with highly salted and seasoned foods, condiments, coffee, tea and liquor are continually being sexually stimulated by these foods. I have heard these claims for many years. Just what foundation or basis there is for these claims I cannot state. While they contend that these foods do stimulate the sexual desires and act like an aphrodisiac, they also cause the same people to lose their virility at an early age.

Their contention may have some sound basis for they claim the above foods cause irritation in the genital organs which is to a certain degree stimulating to the sexual desires ... but there is also the long range effect of setting up complications and troubles in the urogenital area.

One authority whom I esteem quite highly makes the claim that consumption of these foods irritates the urogenital tract and is a contributing cause of premature ejaculation. He goes further and claims that more than 50% of all males have this problem.

Many people are of the opinion or have been led to believe that vegetarianism is a safe and sure way to avoid or prevent prostate conditions. Many people believe that vegetarians do not suffer from urinary and prostatate malfunctions.

It is my contention that this is purely wishful thinking among vegetarians and there is no truth to the belief that vegetarians do not have troubles with their genital and urinary organs. My experience indicates that they have almost as many of these troubles as the conventional or meat-eating people.

However, among people who follow the strict hygienic way of life and who do not use salt or chemically treated foods and whose diets consist mainly of unfired foods, there is, to the best of my belief, a very low or non-existent incidence of prostate conditions. Of course, I mean among those who have been following this way of life for many years. In most cases, however, the followers of the hygienic or vegetarian way of life are usually men who, because of illness or other circumstances were forced to adopt this method, usually later in life, and therefore they cannot be cited as examples.

I do not know of any instances where children or even young people started on the hygienic or vegetarian way of life and have followed it religiously. Therefore I cannot say whether or not they could avoid prostate disorders in this manner.

However, my inquiries among vegetarians do not indicate that they are immune to prostate troubles. In fact, I have reached the conclusion that they do have prostate troubles to varying degrees. It would appear from my inquiries that they do not have as high an incidence of prostate trouble as do conventional eaters. Nevertheless I want to stress that vegetarianism is not necessarily a positive way to avoid prostate disease.

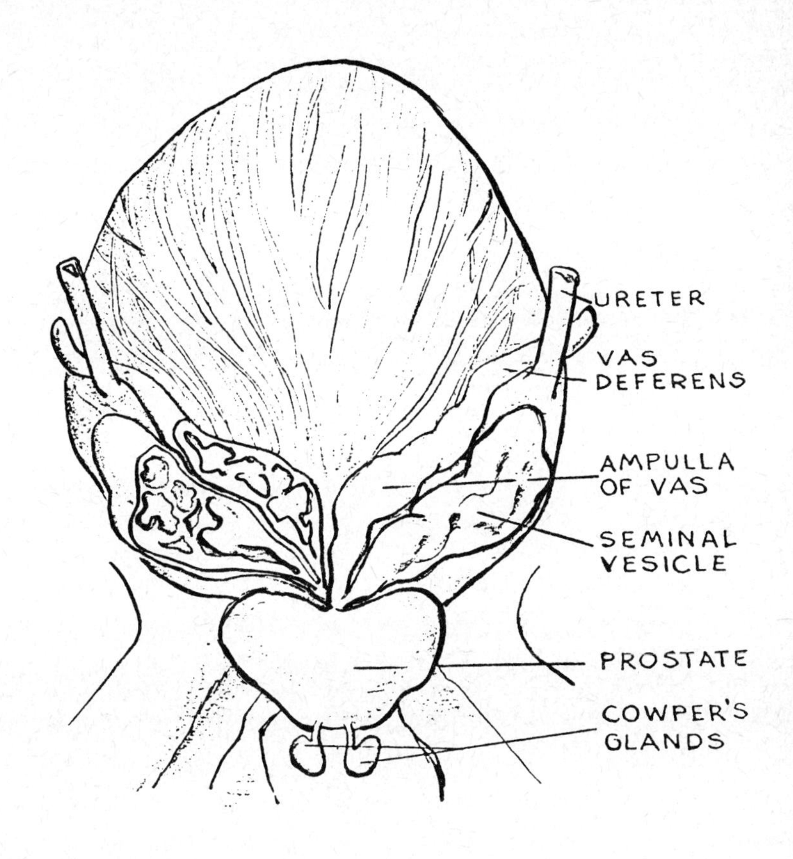

DISTENDED BLADDER, SEMINAL VESICLES, PROSTATE AND COWPER'S GLANDS AS SEEN FROM BEHIND

SEMINAL VESICLES

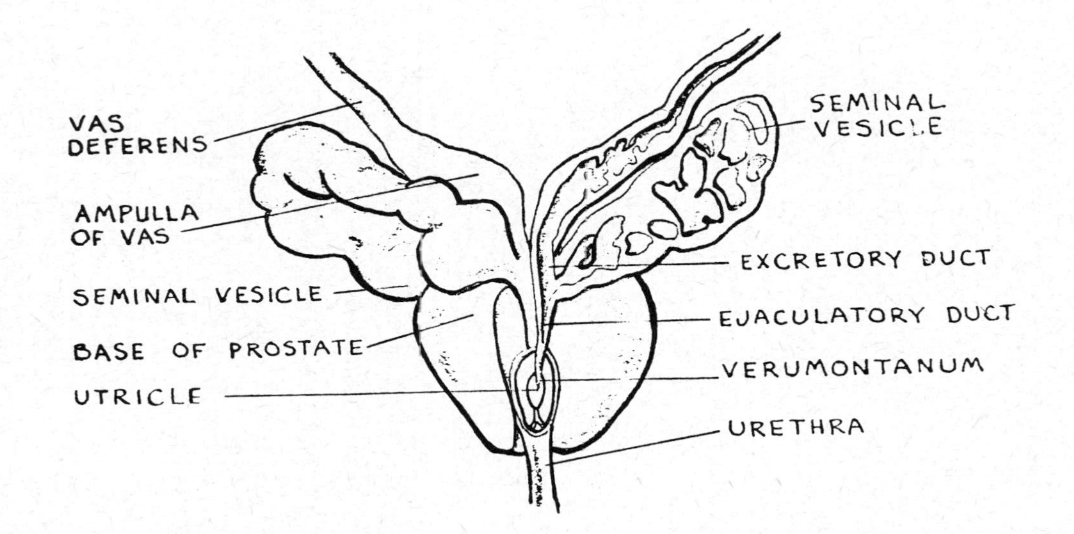

Chapter Nine

SEX AND YOUR PROSTATE

You or some people or even the critics may say that this is a book mainly about sex. I will stoutly deny that suggestion. This book is on the prostate from start to finish. However, the prostate is the sex gland ... so sex must be our focal point in so far as it affects the prostate.

In my sober moments, as I reflect, it is undeniable the magnitude of the vital role that sex plays in the lives of men and women and especially in men. It would be no joke or exaggeration if I said that the whole world revolved around the sexual organs of a man and a woman.

I know that some people -- especially those in advanced years who have no interest in normal sex relations -- will rise quickly and deny the validity of my statements but that makes little difference to me. They can deny it from now till doomsday but the fact still emerges and is known that the world does revolve on the genital organs of men and women.

All other considerations are secondary.

Life, religion, well-being, health, happiness, wealth, whether they be on different levels or positions, all run second to sex. Without the sexual capacity in the male there can be no motivation, no bodily, mental or physical strength. The regular partaking of sexual activity governs all of the potentials of a human being.

A man may lead an exemplary life -- he may eat of the best foods in the land -- he may even eat of the fat of the land -- he may be wined and dined -- he may be groomed and burnished -- he may work and have exercise -- he may study and learn -- he may be a lord or a pauper -- but all is not well with him unless he has a normal sex life.

When in a human being the need for sex arises and sometimes this happens in a youth without his recognizing or realizing that it is sex that he needs, he can neither work nor study nor play. His appetite fails, he is unable to think rationally, he doesn't know what is wrong with him ... but sexual satisfaction can, in practically every case, correct all of these faults. To put the situation in its stark bold light, a man's intellect cannot function correctly or at its best while he has an erection. Not until that erection is relieved can his body return to normalcy.

Long before reaching this chapter you will no doubt have recognized the true simple fact that no one -- scientist, healer, practitioner, sociologist, researcher, urologist or layman -- knows much about the prostate or the male genital organs in general. It seems that for all the multi-millions of dollars at their disposal, neither the scientists, the healers nor the government can find out just what it is that makes the human being tick.

Since childhood I have observed, read, studied, questioned and experienced many and varied things concerning sex and the sex organs. Even at the risk of sounding like a braggart, I sincerely believe that I have as much knowledge concerning this part of the human body as most people -- even the so-called experts. Yet I admit that when it comes down to basic, sound, fundamental, intricate functions, I know little or nothing -- just like the experts.

Now to start with, I'd say that I have found that sex is absolutely essential for the normal development, health and longevity of the normal human being. On the other hand, there are eminent authorities who claim that a human being can live a normal life in perfect health and well-being without sex. They probably can defend their position as well or better than I. So let's put it this way ... Those who do not require sex themselves think and believe and go out of their way to prove that sex is unnecessary. Those, like myself, who find sex necessary and important in their lives go all out to prove that sexual relations are not only necessary but vital for sound health and long life.

Most authorities maintain that practically all of the difficulties, abnormalities and problems connected with prostatic disturbances, are in some way attributable to sex and its various practices. I, for one, do not accept the theory that sexual activity is the main cause of prostatic derangement. It is my sincere belief that there are many factors involved and that sexual activity is only a part, be it lesser or greater.

The total sum of all the knowledge that I have gleaned (and I have not yet stopped digging for information, even at the time this book is going to press) conclusively accentuates the fact that normal or regular sexual relations are definitely not a causative or provocative or contributory factor in prostate disease. It is known and understood that a physically and mentally healthy human being requires sexual relationship and that it should be a regular practice with every normal man. But it should be indulged in only after prescribed or understandable foreplay or love-making.

First of all sex is probably the greatest and most pleasing sensation to which a human being can hope to aspire. Anyone who does not subscribe to this belief is either a moron, a sexual pervert, a homosexual or a decrepit old man or a frigid woman.

I do not suggest or advocate excesses however ... but who is to judge what is and what is not "excess"? Sexual intercourse should be indulged in as the need and the desire manifest themselves and of course it should be indulged in, wherever possible, with a lawfully wedded mate. Thus, if it is indulged in as desired -- and the body is able and willing -- is there such a thing as "excess"? I furthermore consider that being aroused sexually to varying heights or degrees and then being frustrated can and will cause serious harm to the human anatomy. I believe that this is also a strong contributing factor to prostatic disease.

It is my belief that deviations from what is generally accepted and known as regular, properly practised sexual intercourse are the greatest cause of sexual impotency.

I do not advocate or suggest the use of any form of artificial stimulation. Obviously there are various nefarious ways in which this may be achieved but I know no method that is advisable, practical or safe. I have been told, I have read, I have learned that there are herbs, drugs and even mechanical devices that can be used to create desire ... but I sincerely suggest to my readers that they take no part in any of these maneuvers. If you will maintain or build good health, then you will be able to participate in sex with normal frequency and in a normal manner without any aphrodisiacs of any kind.

I recall something that I learned from reading a volume on eugenics when I was a mere youth. I don't remember the author's name now. However, he stated that the mucus-like, oily substance that is emitted through the penis when one is aroused sexually or while indulging in love-making is a provision on the part of nature to prepare the organ for the actual sexual relationship. In this treatise, the author, a man of wide experience, claimed that if one had sexual relations without waiting for this flow to pave the way it could be a contributing factor to sexual organ disturbances. The author further claimed that continued violation or abuse of this nature would ultimately result in lost manhood.

A bit of reflection will clearly indicate that nature does nothing needlessly or without a definite purpose and if it were her intent to prepare the organ for a specific function, then the act should not be consummated until nature has performed her preliminary task.

If you have taken the time to observe animals' actions before, during and after sex, you will have seen quite a different performance to that practised by man in our civilized and accepted way of life. With animals all goes according to a predetermined pattern and there are no aberrations.

Human beings are supposedly superior animals. They can and do perform the sex act from calm to climax in a matter of an hour or a few minutes or a few seconds, as the situation demands. As you know, human beings are always in a heck of a hurry about anything, something or nothing ... to do one thing or another and go somewhere, elsewhere or nowhere. So even when it comes to something as paradisiacal as sexual intercourse, in most cases they don't have time to wait until nature completes her essential preparatory work.

Then, too, it must be admitted that the sex act is often performed clandestinely. I am not moralizing in this instance. I am neither condemning nor condoning -- I am simply relating facts. Therefore, being done clandestinely, this would often necessitate a great deal of subterfuge, stealth and hurry. In such instances nature would, of course, be circumvented in her prescribed purpose.

Now whether or not the failure to wait for this normal preparatory organic function to take place is a factor in bringing about prostatic trouble, I do not know. I maintain that no one knows for certain. But I state as my opinion that this "failure to wait" is a strong contributing factor in malfunction of the prostate. Furthermore, I believe it is my duty to bring this important matter to your attention. I would strongly urge every male who reads this book to follow nature's scheme of things to the letter and wait until she gives you the green light.

If you have not properly prepared yourself for the consummation of the sexual act, due to shyness, debility, lack of knowledge or other causes, I urge you to start at once to acquire this vital knowledge and adopt such measures so that you may forestall impending serious trouble with your sexual organs ... especially with your prostate.

I would like to issue a stern warning. Failure to complete the act or obtain full gratification will definitely create a blocking and congestion of the prostate and the seminal vesicles. This can and does result in harm to the anatomy. This vital bit of information is a little bit of detail that some writers and authorities forget or ignore.

I further stress that when you allow yourself to be aroused sexually, you should try by all normal proper means to carry out nature's intent by fulfillment, which means sexual communion.

One must learn the difference between an erection due to sexual desire and an erection due to an overloaded bladder or other irritation of the genitals. Actually I am sure the average individual knows the difference but some make use of any erection for the practice of sexual relations. Do not attempt to perform the sex act with an erection that is due to bladder distention for it can result in serious harm to your bladder, to your kidneys and to your prostate. The proper course to follow is to first empty the bladder and then, if you are still in the mood for sexual relationship, it is quite proper to indulge in the act.

Just how masturbation affects the prostate I am not able to state, nor can I find any information on the subject from all the sources which I have investigated. However, it must be recognized, whether we approve or not, that the practice of masturbation is widespread. Of course many people can understand such happenings among young boys but fail to recognize that it is widely practised among adults.

Masturbation is also known as narcissism and the dictionary would explain this by saying it was excessive self-love or self-love-making. According to Kinsey's Report 93% of all males have indulged in or practised masturbation at some period in their lives.

Only 58% of all females fit into this category. It appears that masturbation appeals mostly to those at the age of puberty when a sexual relationship between the two sexes is not generally available or practical for any number of reasons which are best known to the individual himself. Therefore, masturbation is the end result of our civilized way of life.

The generally accepted views concerning masturbation have always mystified me. Please let me explain ... I have always believed masturbation to be a heinous, harmful, vile, vicious practice that was indulged in by a small deranged segment of our society. But to my disgust and amazement I learned that it is so widely condoned by some as to reach the point of tacit acquiescence or approval. Perhaps this is due to thinking in terms of 'let who is without sin among ye cast the first stone.' I am most strongly opposed to that kind of thinking and I still maintain that masturbation is most unnatural and vicious, no matter how widely it is practised. Besides, in my opinion, it is degrading. However, irrespective of my views, it must be examined in its right and proper perspective.

Consider the position of any normal male being who desires sexual gratification and is unable, because of any one of many reasons including convention and circumstances, to find satisfaction. Among these are sailors, prisoners and convicts, as well as men who because of duty are away from women for extended periods of time. Then who has the right among us to stand up and say that he is perverted because he indulges in the only form of gratification that he knows? I do not under any circumstances condone the practice -- I condemn it -- but I also accept the cold fact that it is broadly practised. In truth, nature provides an escape or an outlet for such circumstances by promoting a nocturnal emission when the body and mind require it.

Why an emission brought about by masturbation should be any more harmful to the prostate than an emission brought about by sexual intercourse I cannot tell. Not having practised this act (masturbation) I cannot speak with the voice of authority. In truth, I don't even have a clue, unless it results in forcing or over-exertion which normal coitus should not. But who knows ... masturbation may not be forcing or over-exerting. Nevertheless it is widely accepted by many authorities that masturbation contributes in a marked degree towards prostatic hypertrophy.

Sometimes the sudden loss of the female partner brings about cessation of sexual activity. This might happen to a normal man who has, in the course of his married life, indulged in sexual relationship regularly over a period of many years. Suddenly his sex life is brought to an abrupt end and if he is of a retiring disposition, a new contact is not established. I would consider it a serious matter if the male partner does not have sexual relationship for a matter of years or even months. It might cause serious harm to the prostate. This is not a very frequent occurrence but nevertheless it can be a contributor to prostatic disorders for such men.

Now I would like to deal with another phase and that is the ardent male who has a cool or frigid spouse.

I have been acquainted with a few men in such circumstances. It literally means that this man goes around in an almost continual state of desire. Some men in such circumstances will find extra-marital partners. Then there are many who do not commit adultery for religious or moral or other reasons. This frustration, continued over a period of years, must lead to serious prostatic trouble. I am not attempting to pass on advice to such unfortunate males but I know what it must mean to their peace of mind -- besides the serious harmful effect it may have on their prostate. But don't ask me and quote me when it comes to counselling men who find themselves in this predicament.

It is my contention that when this natural sexual urge must be continually repressed, it is dangerous. In fact, I would say it is not only dangerous to the prostate but to the entire nervous system as well. I sincerely believe that the moral or legal code or law should provide an outlet for an unfortunate male who finds himself in this predicament.

It is further my belief that to restrict a male under such circumstances because of social mores or other restrictions, be they religious, financial or otherwise, places a tremendous burden upon a poor, ordinary, normal human being. If you were to tell me that such men become lunatics and go stark raving mad, I would understand it. It is not right in any sense of the word or by any code to deprive a man of his natural and normal functions.

Many men do not accept such restrictions, but there are men of the highest cultural and moral standards who do ... and for these men I have great sympathy and understanding.

Now a moment on 'nocturnal emission', which is also referred to as 'night loss', 'wet dreams', 'nocturnal pollution' even, as some purists refer to it, or 'onanism' ... although I believe this is stretching a point. This is a natural procedure, one that I believe the body uses to prevent the clogging up or harming of the prostate and other essential organs. This is something over which a youth or any unmarried man has very little or no control. It should not occur in the life of a married man unless he is parted from his wife for some reason. When nature commands the occurrence takes place, with or without his consent. I don't think this can be held against the youth and cannot in any way be compared with masturbation or onanism.

Some men, I understand, find these nocturnal emissions distasteful and are somewhat worried about them. My own thought on the subject is that they are not to be feared but to be accepted or actually welcomed, like any other normal function of the human body.

However, when a married man has a nocturnal emission, something is radically wrong ... unless due to an enforced separation from his wife. It would indicate that he is having insufficient sexual relations and this condition should be remedied. Nature is telling him in no uncertain terms that this stored up seminal and glandular fluid needs to be ejected and, under the circumstances, a nocturnal emission is normal and to be expected.

Among males who find regular sexual gratification I doubt if nocturnal emissions occur, except on rare occasions. I realize that among men in advanced years this type of thing may not be welcome. On the other hand, I have a second thought on the matter and I think the older man should regard himself as fortunate because this manifestation proves he is still sexually healthy and virile and he need feel neither shame nor guilt, for actually it is neither a sign of weakness nor pollution.

As the years advance women find less need for sex and the male partner as a rule must learn to resign himself to such curtailment. On the other hand, many men do not accept this restriction of what they deem to be their rightful pleasure or liberty and they clandestinely find themselves mistresses or visit prostitutes.

Please bear in mind that male and female sexual physiology are at great variance. Since a woman does not have a prostate gland or seminal vesicles, when she no longer feels the sex urge, it does not seriously affect either her mental or physical well-being. Therefore, I would suggest that the moral code that applies to a woman does not necessarily apply to a man. It must be remembered that in the male organs, in the prostate and correlated organs presumably, the ducts that house the sperm fill up automatically and do become overloaded and if this accumulation is not discharged at regular intervals, harm -- serious or otherwise -- can result ... and this may be another important contributor to prostate troubles.

In the Orient and among Moslems, men are allowed concubines, or several wives. Perhaps in this way they avoid this one specific contributing factor in prostate disorders.

A spontaneous emission, when brought about by normal sexual relations, will drain the prostate gland as well as the seminal vesicles completely, properly and conveniently. By means of this emission the glands are exercised and retain their tone and resiliency. It must be recognized that if the prostate, the seminal vesicles and all of the sexual glands are not put to their intended use when the need arises or if they are left to stagnate for months or years, trouble will no doubt ensue and the prostate gland will be harmed.

It is my opinion that from youth to middle age a man in good health should require sexual indulgence from three to seven times a week. However, I know that there are many males in the same age category in this present day and age who do not indulge in sexual intercourse more than once or twice a month. This, I suggest, is a very poor average and there is something radically wrong with a man in his youth or middle age who cannot perform or does not desire the sexual act at least every other day. Furthermore, I maintain that this average should be maintained by a normal, healthy man into his sixties. Whether you wish to accept this or not, I stoutly maintain that it is true and I believe that I can defend my position.

It is, however, generally recognized that man's sexual potency begins to wane in his 40's or at the best, in his 50's. Men who perform the act every day in their 20's often get down to 5 times a week in their 30's and every other day in their 40's and in their 50's it varies from once to twice weekly. Then in their 60's it drops to once or twice monthly. Now when I said weekly I meant ever seven days, although in many cases it is correctly spelled weakly.

The decline in sexual activities is not always an indication that something is wrong with the prostate. I contend that often a nutritional problem is involved and that the overall health picture is not good. It is easy to understand that if the overall health picture is poor, the libido is sure to suffer. In fact, it is one of the first bodily functions to suffer.

I am sure you all know that a thin man is better prepared for sexual activity than a stout man. Obesity is usually a definite indicator that the individual is not sexually strong. It is invariably the slight men who perform better sexually. Obese men seldom, if ever, have the sexual potency or the virility of their thin brothers.

My inquiries reveal that sexual failures at 40 are quite common. I have checked in a great number of cases and was amazed, alarmed, astounded to learn that many men of 40 indulge in sexual relations only once or twice a month. This should not be. A healthy male should be able to perform the sex act at least every other day at the age of 40 to 50 ... at least, in my opinion. If you cannot perform the sex act that frequently at that age I would suggest that you quickly look into the matter of the state of your health. Kinsey in his work on sexual incidence rates two to three times weekly for the average male of 40 years of age.

Another theory that I would like to explode is the one that because you indulged frequently in sex when you were young you used up your energies and therefore you can expect to be impotent or weak sexually in your middle and old age.

There is a school of thought that maintains that every male human has only so many orgasms in him and when these are used up, well, that's it. So they advise caution and abstinence or restraint in youth.

That is absolutely wrong. Those who have had much intercourse in their youth should have much as they get older. The lessening should be proportional. A strong, virile youth usually means a strong, virile middle and old age. So don't be misled into believing that a sexually vigorous youth means anything less than a sexually vigorous middle and old age ... if you are intelligent enough to retain your health.

There are men or, at least, there were men -- I don't know if they exist today -- who performed the sexual act daily throughout their entire reproductive lifetime ... yes, until they were 60 and even 70 years of age ... and they did not suffer one iota from lack of energy. Most of the sexually active men that I have known during my lifetime had more vigor into old age than did the sexually inactive men.

I am thinking of an individual I knew very, very well who claimed that he had performed the act at least every day until the time he was past 70 years of age. I recall saying to him, "Why, this is ridiculous! You can't have intercourse with your wife every day. What about the times when she menstruates?"

His reply was, "I said that I had intercourse every single day and I meant what I said. Do you want me to draw you a picture? Furthermore, I intend to maintain this pace as long as I live."

I did not press the point further.

This man died in his early seventies but I don't think death was due to over-indulgence in sex. I would like to add that this man worked hard physically and led a very active life.

I beg of you to evaluate the facts concerning sexual frequency. Check up for yourself and you will learn that I do speak the truth. Therefore, do not think to husband your strength and your energy by restricting your sexual output. I maintain that it is false economy. It is now known that periodic discharge of the semen has a positive stimulating effect upon both the mind and the body. Instead of draining the vitality from the body it promotes initiative and vitality. It is positively established and generally accepted that virile, sexually active men live longer than celibates and eunuchs.

Of all the creatures on earth man is the only one who practises various forms of sexual abnormalities or anomalies. These deviations from the norm take on a range of ways and means in wide scope. In animals the sexual practice is more or less fixed and follows a routine pattern without digression.

It is known that all animals perform the sex act as the call arises and as nature directs when they meet or seek out opposite members of their species. Man, however, performs the sex act as convention and circumstances decree and he must rise to the occasion like a trained, harassed animal. Man does not always have the privilege of performing the sex act when he is in the mood or when it strikes his fancy. To make matters more complicated, there are so many inhibitions, taboos, rules, regulations and other infringements concerning sex that I proclaim it is the most disturbed, disrupted, unharmonious and deflected of all the essential corporeal functions performed by a human being.

On top of all this, he or his spouse has to worry about pregnancy, venereal diseases, being seen or caught or disgraced or other predicaments that surround the performance of this most essential and necessary function. You may say that when sex is indulged in by a couple who are married, these factors do not enter into it but I will remind you that even married folk cannot perform the sex act whenever they have the urge or when the passions are aroused. Remember, they are bound by rules, regulations, mores and conventions, too. For example, the children may be present, friends may be in attendance, they may be in company, they may be out visiting. Yet no one has particular control over the rise and fall of the sex urge and if the desire comes upon one under certain circumstances, one just does not indulge, because civilization has taught us to develop proper control. But please remember that this does not occur with any other animal but the human.

The average man, in order to indulge in sex, often has to coax, tease, cajole and practise intrigue, sculduggery, sneaking machiavellian tactics and other sub rosa practices to procure his sexual relations. Often he has to run after it, hunt it, trap it and be ready to indulge whenever the opportunity, the circumstances and the female will allow.

No one can deny that the back seat of a parked car in lover's lane is not the most desirable, conducive or suitable place in which to perform the sex act, yet it is performed as often under such circumstances as it is in a bed -- at least, in America.

Furthermore, the man must produce the erection and maintain it as long as the female desires it. He is but a performer, an actor or a clown or a trained seal and he must do it to please or else have his opportunities seriously curtailed.

Just how big or important a part these antics and gyrations play in the cause of prostatic disorders I do not know but I would suggest that these outlined maneuvers play a most important part in the degeneration of the prostate gland.

Often couples will enjoin in long bouts of petting because the opportunity for sexual fulfillment has been denied them for any one of a great number of reasons. This sustained erection and sexual excitement can and does wreak havoc with a man's anatomy and his nervous system as well as his prostate. This matter is worthy of deeper thought and consideration.

It is generally agreed by practitioners that the sexual symptoms that go along with prostatic disease are so varied and numerous that it would be a major undertaking to classify all of them.

It is maintained by some of the best authorities that impotency is caused more frequently by disturbed prostate than by any other condition. While certain symptoms point directly to the prostate, there may be many symptoms that could involve many other organs or be caused by different maladies.

There is a condition frequently found in men of all ages known as precipitancy or premature ejaculation or "coitus praecox." In simple terminology it means that finis is written to the sexual act before it is commenced or immediately following the penetration into the vulva. In some circles a sexual encounter of less than fifteen minutes duration might be referred to as coitus praecox. Then again any bout of sexual intercourse that fails to allow sufficient time for the female partner's climax might be called coitus praecox. Another interpretation of coitus praecox is ejaculation even before the penis has penetrated the vulva or vagina. However, my interpretation of coitus praecox would be any ejaculation by the male that was involuntary or uncontrollable.

Whether this condition has any connection or relationship with the prostate or prostate enlargement I am unable to say, but this condition is definitely found to exist among many males and some authorities echo the belief that it is caused by prostate disorders.

Whenever something is amiss with the sexual or genital organs, a study of the prostate should be made immediately.

Elsewhere in this book I pointed out that man, of all the creatures on the face of the earth, is the only one that practises sex 365 days a year and most frequently for other reasons than propagation. Furthermore, it is invariably the female and not the male who decides whether or not sexual intercourse will take place. This certainly places the female in an enviable position of authority.

Of course, there's the exception of out and out rape. However, because I know my fellow man and also a wee bit about women, I have learned that many women, even if they do not desire the sex act for themselves, will condescend to give their bodies to their mates for any one of many reasons. It could be for love, it could be for money, it could be for gifts, it could be out of the goodness of their hearts, it could be for pity ... but the fact is that among all the creatures on earth only the human female will permit sex even if the inherent desire does not exist within her.

Please give close attention to this phase of my argument. I am sure that you have seen female dogs and cats, and perhaps other animals, viciously repel the male when he sought to indulge in sex outside of the mating or rutting season. I have known them to be so vicious and aroused that they have killed the male for attempting copulation. However, with the human female, even though she is not in the mood, even though she does not need it, even though she does not want it, she will, if she is in a condescending mood, allow sexual relations. I say again that this does not take place with any other creature or being on earth.

Let us now get back to our situation. Does this overworking of the prostate by comparatively regular sexual congress, unlike any other creature, contribute to the destruction of the prostate? I would say, yes. It is my belief that it was never intended that man partake of or indulge in sex throughout the entire calendar year. This one significant factor may be the prime cause of or contributor to prostate disorders.

On the other hand, I devoted a part of this book to telling you that men who rarely or seldom indulge also have prostate troubles. So there we are. Where are we? Up a tree! I point out a very significant factor and then by other examples, I negate it. Do you wonder what kind or manner of man I am? The truth of the matter is, I did not set out to prove anything when I began to write this book. I am just trying to present the facts in their true light.

Now let me deal with another facet of this intriguing situation. No one can deny that emotional factors enter into the pattern of behaviour of human beings. Fidelity, love, desire, jealousy, passion, attraction, coquetry, hate and such feelings affect the mental stability of humans whereas this phase is insignificant or of minor importance in other animals. But anyone who has made any study whatsoever of the prostate and the factors involved must have reached the conclusion that somewhere along the line the emotions and the prostate seem to have a very close link. Whether the prostate contributes to the emotional upsets or whether the emotional upsets affect the prostate, I am unable to say, but I am convinced that there is a definite co-relation between them. May I, at this time, suggest that men who have frequent or continual emotional upsets or problems are men who do or will suffer prostate problems? Therefore, it is an axiom, I maintain, that if one wishes to be free of prostate disorders, he seek to maintain emotional balance or equilibrium.

They claim that, when seeking the pleasures of sex, one invariably goes overboard. Well, it is characteristic of human beings to go overboard and over-indulge in many things and I don't see why sex should be an exception. Perhaps because of frustrations, because of problems, because of difficulties, especially those concerned with the amenities of life in our present civilization, one seeks to find pleasure where one may ... and who would or could deny them that right? Sex, being so close and so handy and so pleasureful, is a marvelous outlet. Evidently, here again, no other creatures on earth have to seek this indulgence as a mode of escape.

Then the matter of sexual knowledge comes into the picture. Do the average young man and woman know enough about their sex organs, the sex act and the ultimate outcome to allow them to be the judge of the advisability of what they are doing? Frequently throughout my lifetime I have come across men and women who in a short discussion concerning marriage and sex, appalled me by their abyssmal ignorance of what I would call vital matters that pertained to the well-being of the man, the woman and the children.

For example, it is generally believed and accepted that sexual intercourse is not to be indulged in during the menstrual period. One of the first rules and regulations outlawing sexual relations during this period was laid down by the Jews four or five thousand years ago. I think that was the first reference ever made and the first rule covering this situation. Yet today, medical science claims that they see no rhyme or reason why sex cannot be indulged in during the menses. Now please do not misunderstand me ... I am not advocating relations at that period. I am only stating this for your information.

Let's take another example. How many couples of any age know that conception rarely takes place while the mother is breast-feeding an infant, even if the breast-feeding extends to eighteen months or even beyond two years? How many couples know or understand that sex should not be indulged in at the drop of a hat but that it should be led up to by proper love-making and foreplay?

I could go on and cite, I am sure, a hundred different examples and each would indicate that few people really understand the truth about sex and sexual relations. To the best of my knowledge I know of no institution or department that gives full or complete instructions concerning sexual relations. This most important part of the lives of human beings is conducted haphazardly, catch-as-catch-can. Is it any wonder that we have emotional and prostate and other troubles?

Just how important a role do civilization's controls, inhibitions, rules, laws, regulations, moral codes and human decency play in the root of our prostate troubles?

Please forgive me for making the continued reference to animals but I have nowhere else to turn, especially in dealing with any problem of a biological nature. In the lives of animals none -- not one single one -- of the above factors has any place in or effect upon their way of life. They have no inhibitions, rules, regulations or moral codes by which they must live. Sexual relations are something that take place as demand or need or circumstances permit. Thus, in these matters they are governed entirely by instinct. Strange to relate, if man followed his instinct in sexual matters, he'd probably find himself in serious trouble. In simple language, I am saying that our natural desires and needs are second fiddlers to convention.

Today throughout the world, but especially in America, we have three sexes -- not two as there used to be. We have males and females, of course, but we also have neuters. They can be of either the male species or the female species -- unlike bees where the neuters are only the undeveloped females.

For some time now I have been trying to decide which specifically is man's strongest or most commanding instinct, desire or need. I asked myself which one of the many ... the desire for food, the wish for money, the quest for fame, the need for happiness, the search for health and long life or the desire for sex or something else? After reading, studying and questioning, I have reached the conclusion that sex is the strongest motivating force in the life of a human being, especially with the male of the species ... although at times the female may reach a pitch of desire that equals or exceeds that of a man.

With many men this sexual desire begins in infancy, reaching a crescendo between the age of puberty and the age of majority. With some men this pinnacle lasts until the 30's and sometimes into the 40's, but seldom beyond. Then, too, I have known many men who have boldly stated that if they could no longer indulge in sex they'd rather be dead.

Well, with an urge as strong as that, one must expect to have complications ... and I suspect that trouble with the prostate is but one of the manifestations.

At some point in my extensive reading about the prostate the thought occurred to me that if it were possible to get records concerning celibates or monks or other males who seldom if ever indulge in sexual relations, this could be a very important indicator concerning the diseases of the prostate. If this data were available, we would know very quickly just how important a part abstinence from sexual intercourse plays in prostatic disorders.

However, an even more important study would be that of the parish priest who in his visits among his parishioners has continuous provocation ... that is, the rising and falling of his emotions continuously by being faced with stimulation without gratification. This is emphatically no reflection on any religion, religious order or group but these are little matters that I would like to know about, if the information were at all available, because they might shed some essential light in reference to the causes of prostatic disorders.

There is another extreme to consider. A cold or frigid wife who restricts a vigorous, healthy, passionate man to once a week or bi-monthly can cause serious trouble of a prostatic nature in the male. But compelling a man who desires or needs sex twice a week to deliver five times a week by a passionate, demanding woman is every bit as bad as an 'every day' man who is restricted to once a week or less.

It is my belief that the man who is cut down too drastically will suffer more than the man who is called upon to perform to a higher degree than his normal desires call for. From such forced abstinence not only does prostatitis develop but it can lead to problems of even a more serious nature. That is, it may turn him into a neurotic, unstable, irrascible, impotent male.

Here is a bit of added proof that sharply focuses attention upon sex relations as the root of prostate trouble. It would appear that the sex act, whether infrequent or frequent, is one of the prime causes of prostate difficulties ... and to add weight or proof to my argument I ask you to consider the fact that it has been discovered that castration invariably reduces the enlarged prostate to normal. As a further clincher ... it is a fact that among eunuchs prostate troubles are absolutely unknown -- they are non-existent.

There is, however, another bit of strange phenomenon involved here because thousands of men develop prostate troubles in their latter years -- the years when their sexual life has come to an end. Now how this can be reconciled with the fact that the sex urge or sex action causes prostate trouble I do not know but it is definitely a fact that men whose sexual life is finished still wind up with prostate trouble. Therefore, even abstinence from sex or impotency still does not prevent a man from having prostate trouble. It is positively recognized that practically all men will develop enlarged prostate if they live long enough.

Chapter Ten

FEAR -- ITS ROLE IN PROSTATE DISORDERS

The shutting off of the urine is, I believe, one of the natural fears to which man is heir. Then because of the high incidence of prostate trouble among males, the cause for fear is strengthened.

I have read of cases among people in remote parts of the world where, when the urinal tract closed up, they resorted to puncturing the abdomen with a pick or knife to permit the urine to escape. In each case death was the result.

I have on occasions (and no doubt so have you) retained my urine for some nonsensical reason like being too busy, too preoccupied, visiting or travelling or such ... and then when at last I had the opportunity to urinate, the flow would not start, at least for some minutes, during which time fear gripped me with an icy vice. When the urine started it was a great relief, though often painful.

Just what part fear plays in prostate disorders or in retention of the urine I don't think anyone can say with any great authority until research along that line has been done, but fear has been known and given as a cause of prostate trouble. Having run the whole gauntlet of prostate trouble, I would like to suggest that fear is of much greater importance than is generally recognized.

My discussions reveal that fear affects the functioning of many bodily organs and definitely among these organs is the prostate. If I had known earlier what I know now and could have eliminated, first and foremost, the fear factor, I am convinced that I could have dealt with the matter in a much more rational and satisfactory manner ... yes, even the ultimate surgery might have been avoided. Yes, questioning and inquiry have revealed that fear appears to be associated with many causes of retention of the urine. For example, fear is definitely known to cause stricture.

The big question is, "How can fear be eliminated?"

For at least 20 years I had cause to fear eventual prostate trouble. From the first few occasions when I found I had a bit of trouble starting to urinate when I awoke, fear began to set in. I was not intelligent enough to realize that my own stupidity and over-indulgences, coupled with a distended bladder loaded with a saline solution, were the direct cause of my trouble.

In my case the background was, to say the least, discouraging. My father suffered from retention of the urine and prostate trouble, my eldest brother was for years beset with the same affliction and another brother 2 1/2 years my senior was continually in a dither because of his prostate.

Once one gets past 30 he begins to see dark clouds on the prostate horizon. Every male seems to talk about it, caution about it, inquire about it and worry about it. One begins to take note of the frequency and the strength of the stream and if you go to an M.D. for a physical, perhaps for an annual check-up or for an insurance policy, one of the things the M.D. is sure to ask is, "How is your stream?" Or else he bends you over and shoves his finger into your rectum to feel your prostate. Even if you are given a clean bill of health, the fact that he has asked about the stream and felt the prostate gives you cause for concern.

In this way, as we move progressively along, let us say, from the late 30's or early 40's and begin to "enjoy these discomforts," we never bother to stop and think or chide ourselves for the indiscretions, for are not these indiscretions the order of the day and part of our pattern of living? So in spite of the fact that we know something is wrong, we permit ourselves to believe that we are just having a bit of difficulty with our genitals and hope that the trouble will soon pass away. Or we kid ourselves into accepting what in truth is logical ... that we are just getting older. Well, let's be realistic ... these lame excuses that we offer ourselves are neither true nor logical, yet we know from what is transpiring that there is something wrong with the prostate.

If I can do no more for you than alert you to the danger of unwarranted fear I will have achieved a fair share of my goal towards helping my readers. This does not mean that you are to disregard all signs of trouble -- it is but to prevent you from being obsessed with unwarranted fear. Please believe me, I consider fear to be one of the chief, one of the vital, one of the important factors in prostate disorders. Fear blinds us to the true cause of our trouble. Make no mistake, fear itself is a most distressing condition to the entire nervous system and again there is a link with the prostate.

Therefore, I suggest that at the first sign of a disorder in that area you deal with the matter rationally and sensibly and face up to it and under no circumstances allow fear to grip you with its harmful hand. Once you permit fear to take hold of you the ultimate result is a foregone conclusion... mental distress, prostate troubles, various treatments and surgery.

Let us deal for a moment with the implications involved in getting up at night to urinate. It is given everywhere as a strong indication that there is something wrong with your prostate.

In this day and age the copious drinking of tea, coffee, beer and other alcoholic beverages is the order of the day. Everybody, but everybody, drinks copious quantities of one or many of the above beverages. You don't have to be a mathematician or statistician to recognize the truth of what I say because the sales of these products are soaring yearly without even a sign of diminishing. I read statistics regularly ...

and coffee sales, tea sales, beer sales, liquor sales and soft drink sales go up and up each and every year.

Well, if you drink excessive amounts of any of these or other beverages, it follows that this fluid will have to be excreted. The chief means of excreting water is through the bladder. It takes approximately four hours for a fluid taken into the body to be filtered through the kidneys and excreted. Therefore, any amount of fluid that is taken into the body a few hours before retiring is naturally a positive factor in rising during the night. It is even more marked as we grow older.

As you have learned elsewhere in this book, the bladder can comfortably hold anywhere from 10 to 16 ounces of fluid. The average bottle of beer contains 12 fluid ounces. The average cup of tea or coffee contains from 6 to 8 fluid ounces. Therefore, the number of cups of tea or glasses of beer or liquor or water that one drinks during the evening will govern the number of times he will have to rise during the night to empty the bladder.

So the fact that you have to get up once or twice during the night does not necessarily indicate that there is something wrong with your bladder or your prostate. It may well be -- in fact, it generally is the true simple fact -- that you have just consumed too much liquid during the evening. So the first test to make for yourself is to try to avoid drinking any fluids after 4 o'clock in the afternoon and then see if you have to get up during the night. Also, avoid partaking of any foods that contain a lot of water after this hour. This experiment must be tried for a few successive nights because a great deal of water is retained by the system in the lymph, blood and practically all body organs and this water too will find its way into your bladder over a period of time. During the day drink only the quantity of water or other liquids the body demands. Avoid all salty foods, condiments, spices, olives, pickles.

Another interesting fact that I'd like to bring to your attention is that salt, especially where used to excess -- and it is found to excess in a normal civilized diet -- can create the impression that there is something wrong with the prostate because excessive salt intake does cause various degrees of irritation, especially in the urethra. Copious amounts of coffee and tea and foods containing chemicals also irritate the genito-urinary tract. This continued irritation can and does eventually cause serious trouble, too, in my opinion.

Here I would like to illustrate a point. If you drink plain, fresh water, it will, in a period of time, have to be excreted and on its way through it will probably pick up varying quantities of salt which will be excreted at the same time. Of course, salt creates its own demand for liquids which cannot be ignored.

If you drink beverages that contain salt (and many beer drinkers put salt in their beer and many coffee makers put salt in their coffee) and eat foods that contain heavy quantities of salt, such as olives, pickles, ketchup, sauces and other condiments, all of the salt thus added has to be excreted. This heavy intake of salt does definitely and positively cause irritation and often a burning sensation as it passes through the urethra. I have learned that large quantities of salt, if consumed regularly, tend to cause a kind of paralysis of the various genital organs. By the avoidance of salt in any form except as found naturally in food, these insidious conditions can be curtailed or completely eliminated.

In many cases fear begins to crop up that we are not urinating sufficiently in relation to our water intake so I'd like to remind you that not all of the water taken into the body is expelled by urination. Remember, water is excreted in the feces, in sweat, in mucus and in tears. Therefore, too much emphasis should not be focused on the amount of fluid eliminated directly by means of urine. Also bear in mind that if you are a heavy salt user, much water is retained in the body until the salt is excreted.

One can very easily measure the intake of water and the amount of water excreted. At one time I was quite concerned about my intake and output and upon measuring I found that there was absolutely no cause for worry because I was voiding reasonably close to the quantity that I was taking in. When you are keeping records, be sure to measure carefully both intake and elimination and they must be measured over at least a 24-hour period.

I am relating this information because I believe it contributes to the fear pattern and by avoiding these offenders you can quickly prove to yourself whether it was your prostate that was causing your trouble or the salt and heavy quantities of liquids that were ingested.

I would suggest that at the first sign of trouble you do not allow yourself to be thrown into a panic. Face up to the situation, reflect upon the cause and reasons for your trouble and analyze it as I suggest. Practise abstinence from harmful drinks and salt for a few days and in some instances the trouble will disappear. This will give you courage and allow you to hold fear at bay. And once you have conquered fear, you are well on your way to conquering prostate troubles in the early stages.

CATHETERS IN PLACE

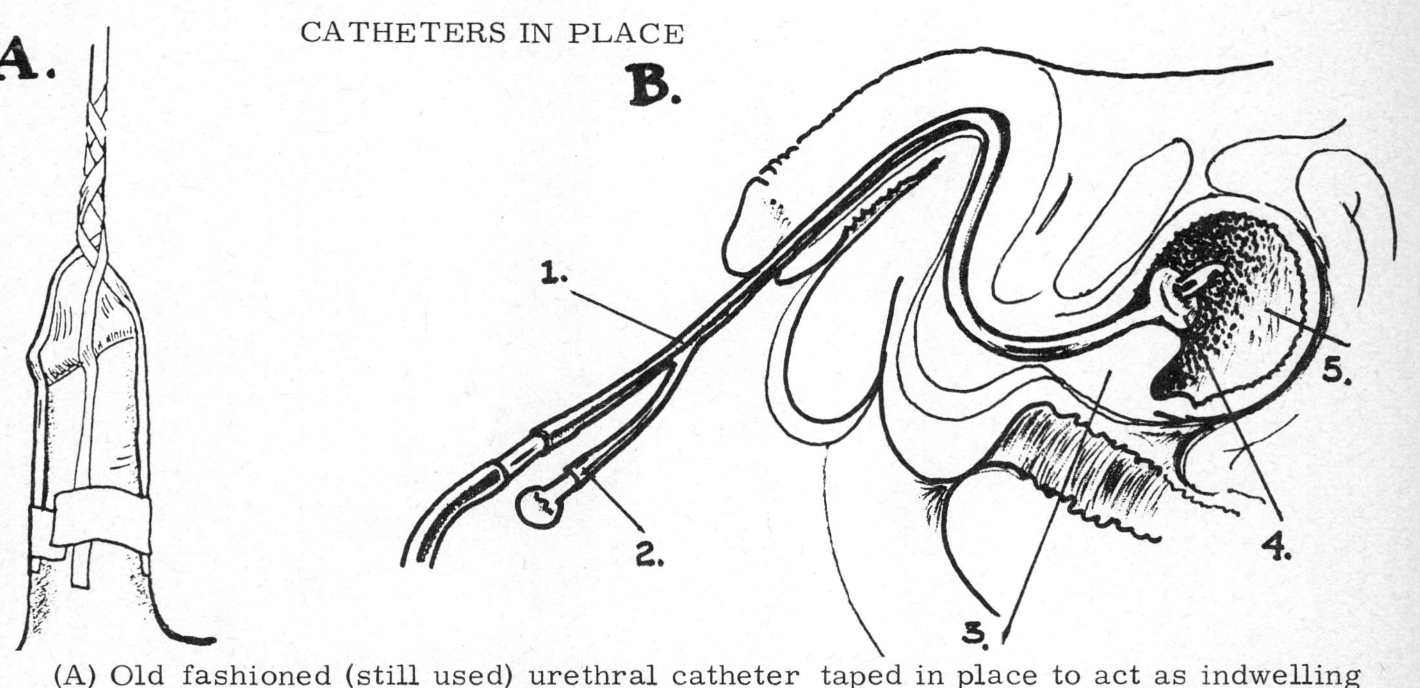

(A) Old fashioned (still used) urethral catheter taped in place to act as indwelling catheter. (B) Indwelling inflatable self-retaining urethral catheter in place. (1) Drainage tube; (2) tube for distention of bag; (3) hypertrophy of prostate; (4) self-retaining bag catheter distended, drawn down to vesicle orifice and resting on vesicle neck.

Chapter Eleven

CATHETERS AND CATHETERIZATION

I tried to learn how long the catheter has been in use. I searched through all the literature available to me and I must tell you that there appears to be practically no information whatsoever on the subject.

The earliest date that I could discover refers to its use as far back as 1622. However, I feel that the catheter must have been used long before that because man must have had trouble with his prostate or bladder from time immemorial. However, there is a possibility, and I will not discount it, that perhaps prostatis or urinary troubles are only of recent vintage and that man's suspicion that prostatic troubles became common when man stopped doing physical labor is gaining strength and is apparently based on solid ground.

Right here near the beginning of this chapter I want to emphasize that catheterization at any time is not child's play. It is to be regarded as a serious, dangerous business and it should never be resorted to unless there is no other means of bringing about urination.

I deliberately focus attention on the dangers of catheterization although to those who are thoroughly experienced in the handling of the catheter it is simple, painless and comparatively without risk. My warning is meant to prevent carelessness on the part of one unskilled in the practice.

Yet I would further warn that even when performed by the most adept professional, eventually, if repeated and repeated, it must lead to disaster. Practically all authorities are agreed that continuous catheterization is always followed by infection and frequently the patient will die from a bilateral pyelonephritis or from a general septicemia, which are infections arising from the urinary tract itself under such abuse.

Catheterization is generally necessary because of inability to urinate and retention of the urine is generally due to some obstruction at or close to the outflow channel. On some occasions it may be due to pressure of swollen glands or a form of paralysis in the surrounding area.

If catheterization is required, I advise that you obtain the services of someone who has had wide experience at performing this work. Some physicians do not have much experience in carrying out this task and seek to avoid it wherever possible. In most hospitals this work is generally relegated to interns and orderlies and that, strictly speaking and man to man, is not good ... for you.

From my understanding, most general

practitioners will avoid injecting a catheter if they can relegate the job to a nurse, an intern or an orderly. They only do it under pressure or serious circumstances. Usually the physician will send you to the hospital and, if necessary, perform it there himself or have someone who he hopes and trusts is proficient in the technique do the job. Usually when one goes to a healer with retention there is no other path open but catheterization. However, it has been my experience that most healers just don't like doing the job.

There are occasions when a catheter cannot be tolerated by a patient with retention of the urine. There are also occasions when a catheter cannot be inserted -- because of obstructions or calculi. Then, too, there are occasions when a catheter is not available.

Under such circumstances other means must be found to empty the bladder. In such cases a trocar is driven into the supra-pubic region just below the umbilicus and above the pubic bone.

In many cases catheterization is a comparatively simple procedure performed by means of a soft rubber or plastic catheter, which is considered the safest, with the least risk of injury to the sexual organ, bladder or prostate. Prior to the invention of rubber and plastic catheters the one commonly used was a silver one ... and because of its solidity, it often caused harm. Good quality catheters can be purchased most reasonably at practically any drug store in America.

After careful reading and observation,

I have found what I believe to be the proper procedure for catheterization, if and when it should be necessary. I will outline it for you and describe the way it is done.

First, the catheter is thoroughly lubricated with a sterile lubricant on the end to be inserted into the urethra through the meatus. The sterile water-soluble jelly makes entrance through the penial aperture comparatively simple. The water-soluble jellies are easier for the system to void than oils of most other kinds. When the catheter has been sterilized and lubricated properly, place yourself on the right side of the patient who is flat on his back with legs spread apart. Take hold of the penis and gently stretch it until it has reached its limit. This is done with the left hand. Then, with the right hand, insert the catheter into the meatus. When this has been accomplished, hold the organ directly upwards.

Then, with the least force possible, slide the catheter carefully into the meatus and into and through the urethra and then slowly inward until it enters the bladder. Do not use force if an obstruction is encountered but try to turn the catheter by revolving it with the fingers, while continuing the forward pressure. In most cases this enables the catheter to slip past any obstruction without using force. With few exceptions this will work and the bladder will be entered without any trouble. When the catheter enters the bladder the flow will commence -- do not force it any further -- and a vessel should be at hand to receive the urine.

It must be clearly understood that urethral shock might occur. This happens more frequently in the aged than in the younger man. This shock, in most instances, is due to the quick emptying of a chronically distended bladder and may cause a fall in blood pressure. In circumstances where one is fearful of the consequences of rapid emptying of the bladder, it can be emptied by drawing only 8 ounces or so off at a time.

From my questioning I learned that there are two distinct schools of thought on the subject of total or partial drainage. One school says to draw off all of the urine and the other says to leave some remaining in the bladder. Personally I don't think that all of the urine will drain off ... specifically because you are usually in a supine position and thus it can't empty completely.

Some urologists and practitioners prefer to leave the catheter in place and not withdraw it until they have established the course of action or treatment to follow. In my discussions with urologists most of them have maintained that there is less danger if the catheter is left in place than in withdrawing and re-inserting it when the need arises.

If there is any belief that the catheter will have to be resorted to frequently, it is far better, in my opinion, to fix it in place and allow it to remain in position for a number of hours or days.

Modern techniques have perfected a catheter for this express purpose. By means of a water bubble which inflates the catheter at one specific point, it can be fixed to remain in position until extraction of the catheter is desired or required. This type of catheter is known as "indwelling" and eliminates the risk of removing and inserting a catheter frequently ... and the subsequent dangers involved.

The catheter, when put in position and attached to a plastic leg urinal, allows the affected person great mobility. In many cases one would never know that there was anything wrong with the patient and he can move about and even travel without any inconvenience or complications.

Please bear in mind that at no time is catheterization any guarantee of recovery or the end of trouble. It is not a cure in any sense -- it is just an expedient. In most cases the necessity of using it is an indication that the trouble is of a serious nature. Therefore, I again stress the fact that catheterization should only be resorted to in extenuating circumstances and should, in every case, be performed by a qualified physician or one who is fully trained in the procedure.

I have known many men who have catheterized themselves frequently without any apparent harm or great distress but, to the best of my knowledge, this is never the solution to the problem. While I submit that it is in many instances a simple procedure, yet catheterization is at best a risky business.

It is not my intention to make you fear catheterization if and when the need arises, nor do I want to give you the idea that it is easy and that you can indulge in it whenever there is an indication of trouble. I am just trying to give you the clear-cut, simple truth concerning the use of this procedure.

Through experience, through reading and through careful study, as well as by inquiry and discussion, I have learned that the average man has an unholy fear of the catheter. I, as a general rule, am not one given greatly to fears or apprehensions, yet I might say that I have been close to being terrified at the thought of ever needing a catheter. It is my sincere belief that I caused myself untold mental stress because I abhored the thought of it and feared to have it used upon me.

I saw my father suffer from a prostate ailment for years and when he eventually had to use a catheter, which incidentally I never saw him do, I was frightfully worried for him. Then I was worried or fearful of the catheter for myself. This fear persisted for most of my lifetime. It was only when I was 57 years old, after going through a lengthy bout with prostatic trouble, that I learned that the catheter could be a valuable friend rather than a deadly enemy.

Please do not misunderstand what I say. I am not telling you that a catheter is good or that you should look forward to the pleasure of using it. It is not any better than a crutch. I am only trying to dispel the fear for the day when you may have to use it ... and this is a grim, but most likely possibility.

If the catheter is handled cleanly, sanitarily, sanely and sensibly, it seldom, if ever, causes complications. It should never be used if you don't need it but when the need does arise, it should be utilized under proper sanitary conditions without qualms or doubts.

NORMAL KIDNEYS

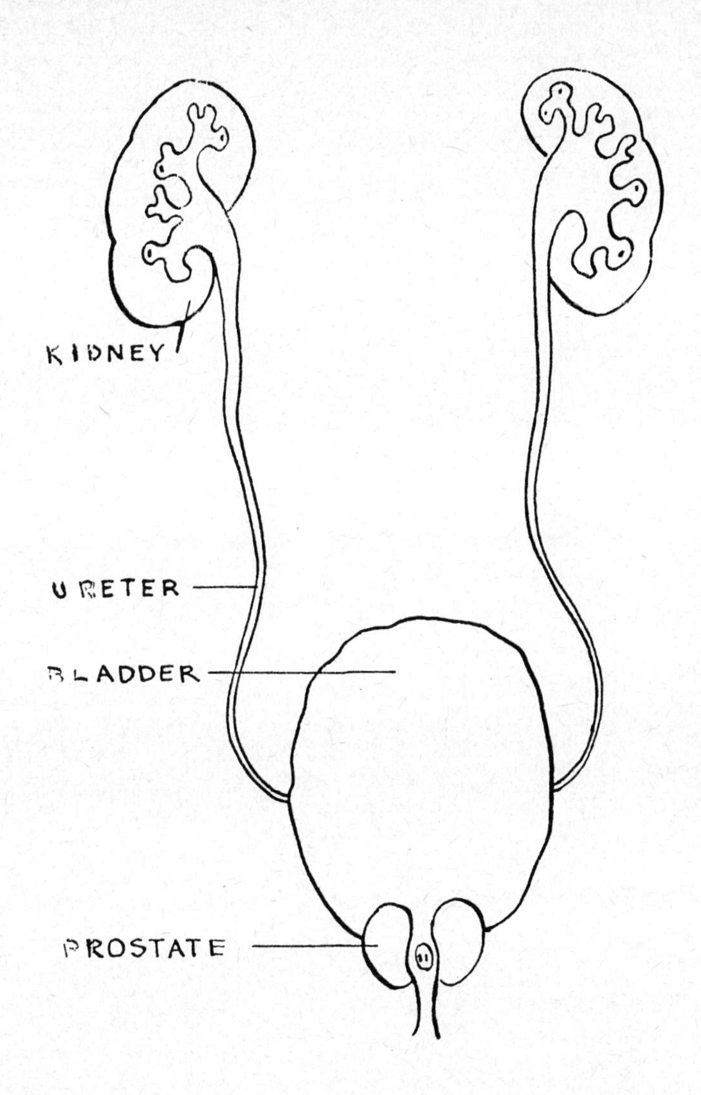

Schematic sketch indicating normal relationship of kidneys, ureters, bladder and prostate.

AFFECTED KIDNEYS

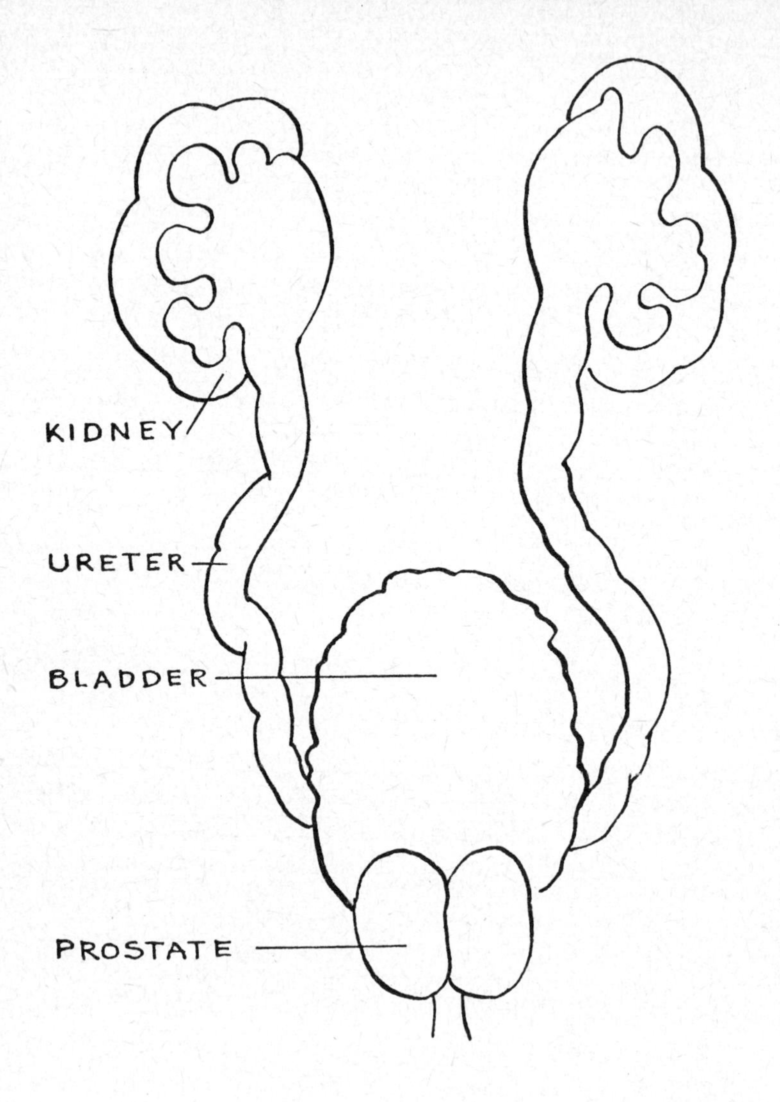

Schematic sketch indicating enlarged prostate and subsequent loss of tone and impaired functional ability of some organs; i.e., kidneys, ureters and bladder.

Chapter Twelve

PREVENTIVE MEASURES

You can avoid or prevent prostate disorders if you follow the rules that I suggest ... and thus you will not only prevent prostate trouble but you will greatly improve the health of your entire body and mind. It will not be easy, but the agony of prostate trouble isn't pleasant either.

1. Drink ample quantities of untreated water.
2. Your diet should consist chiefly, or at least to a large extent, of raw vegetables, fruits, grains and nuts.
3. Avoid all processed, chemically treated foods.
4. Avoid white bread and other bakery products which are loaded with chemicals.
5. Do not use the heavily chemically treated ready-mixes and other bakery products that you have to just pop into the oven.
6. Do not use even home baked products if they contain baking soda or baking

powder or other chemical additives.

7. Avoid fluids after 4 p. m.
8. Avoid any foods containing benzoate of soda or any form of sodium nitrates or sodium nitrites.
9. Eat no canned or processed meat such as corned beef or other spiced meats. They are positively harmful.
10. Avoid salt in any form; that is, added refined salt.
11. Incorporate into your diet in their whole natural form: sesame seeds, flax seeds, sunflower seeds and whole grains cereals.
12. Eat lightly of heavy protein foods such as meat, fish and cheese.
13. Eat no fragmented or devitalized foods.
14. Undergo occasional days of complete abstinence from food.
15. Watch pickles, condiments and other spiced foods. Most contain benzoate of soda and other preservatives.
16. Avoid alcoholic beverages. In excess they are especially dangerous.
17. Urinate promptly in response to nature's call.
18. Take no drugs.
19. Maintain regular, frequent sex relations.
20. Never force the sexual climax.
21. Do not practise masturbation, coitus interruptus, coitus reservatus, or coitus prolongatus.
22. Avoid unduly prolonged sexual stimulus without ejaculation.

23. If your work is sedentary, adopt a regular period for exercise and take frequent long, brisk walks.

Now I expect that the reader will say, "Well, if I have to do all these things and avoid all these other things, life is hardly worthwhile."

I will readily grant that following the above suggestions does make life a bit complicated ... but you will soon find that life will become more meaningful than ever before. I suggest that you bear in mind that nature provided you with a sound organ in the beginning -- at least that is usually true -- and by your living habits you have created this "monster." By formulating the suggestions in this chapter I am only seeking to help you avoid the devastating effects of prostate trouble or to guide and direct you to overcome its ravages.

By following the advice contained herein and avoiding the conditions, habits and foods that bring about these problems, you can, with a fair degree of certainty, prevent this serious malady from striking you and perhaps ruining your life.

Let me ask you this, "Wouldn't it be comforting and worthwhile to know that you are following a way of life that will preserve your good health and your sexual potency up until the time you are in your 7th decade of life and even beyond?"

Yes, I reiterate that by following the advice given in this book your chance of reaching a vigorous, healthful, potent old age can be a reality. Finding a solution to your prostate disorder is of even greater significance when you look about you or take a trip to the old folks' home and see literally hundreds of thousands of men in their 60's and early 70's who have long been impotent and who are doing nothing but vegetating. My conviction is that the foremost underlying contributor to this sad but widespread state of affairs has been diseases or involvements of the prostate.

When measured in the above terms, I am more than certain that you will feel that the rules and advice contained in this chapter are not as restrictive or as Spartan as you first thought they were.

To best illustrate that making these drastic changes in your way of life is worthwhile and not really as hard as it may sound, I'd like to recall to your mind the man who said, "I complained because I had no shoes ... until I saw a man who had no feet."

Chapter Thirteen

RECURRENCE

Perhaps you are under the impression that once you have had prostate surgery your prostate and urinary troubles are over -- for good. Well, I am indeed sincerely sorry to tell you that removing or enucleating your prostate or having a transurethral resection does not necessarily end your urinary and prostate difficulties.

To prove my point I would suggest contacting any ten men at random who have had prostate surgery. Ask them if their problem has been eliminated.

I have interviewed and questioned many men who have had prostate surgery ... and I still do. Some have found complete relief, others partial and some have found that the condition has shown little or no improvement. There were a few who claimed to be actually in worse straits than before.

My further investigations reveal that most complaints emenate from those men who have had transurethral resections of the prostate ... there are more recurrences of prostate trouble by this method. This compels me to sound a warning to those who would seek the easy surgery way out.

Furthermore, in consultation with specialists in internal medicine, I learned that they look with concern upon the transurethral resection method of dealing with the prostate. Contrary to the generally held opinion, the transurethral resection requires greater skill than the other surgical methods.

It is admitted that the perineal and the retro-pubic methods require a great deal of skill, knowledge and experience on the part of the surgeon ... and that is precisely the crux of the situation. Too many surgeons regard the transurethral resection as a cinch, but it isn't a cinch!

I realize that this sounds contradictory and even confusing but you will understand better what I mean when you read the section where these operations are covered in greater detail under "Surgical Treatments."

My informants clearly indicated to me that with the supra-pubic, retro-pubic and perineal, the surgeon is dealing with comparative known factors ... factors which he can see and feel at first hand and can deal with accordingly. With the transurethral he is operating by remote control or at best, indirectly. Therefore, even greater skill, experience and understanding are required.

Furthermore, I am told that greater damage, irreparable damage, can be done by the transurethral than by the other methods.

It is admitted that the transurethral has its advantages ... but I believe it has more disadvantages!

There are many professional men in the various healing fields, including the naturopathic, who will at times admit that it is not possible to clear up advanced prostate troubles without surgery. It must also be recognized that when the condition is far enough advanced even surgery will not perform magic ... especially when cancer is involved. In such cases treatment is not only difficult but frequently in vain.

Many of the healers in the different fields do achieve remarkable results in treatment of the prostate. However, even when they do get results and clear up the trouble, please remember that this trouble can readily recur, especially if your way of life and living and your dietary habits have not undergone a change. If you are fortunate enough to have your troubles clear up by any method of treatment, then I would urge you to quickly change your mode and method of living, drinking and eating.

It is very important to take careful note of the following information regarding recurrence of hypertrophy of the prostate. Most healers in all fields realize that once this abnormality has been allowed to develop, even when it is alleviated or apparently receded or returned to normal, there is a strong possibility of a diathesis for the remainder of the patient's life. By diathesis is meant a built-in constitutional predisposition towards a specific disease.

Even the most hopeful of the practitioners of various schools of healing, apart from the surgical, will tell you that seldom are prostate troubles cleared up so that they will not recur sooner or later. Yes, even when some or all forms of surgery are involved the trouble frequently returns. The usual reason given for this pessimistic note by the healers in such cases is that as we grow older we cannot expect our prostate troubles, or other ailments for that matter, to clear up readily or without repercussions ... and advancing age is cited as being one of the major causes of this trouble.

However, I strictly oppose that line of reasoning. It is my belief, as I have stressed before, that age has little or nothing to do with it, because I have known men of 70 and 80 and well into their 80's who did not have any form of prostate or urinary troubles. Now these men I am referring to are not by any means in great numbers but they do exist, which would clearly indicate to all who care to see that you can live to be 70 or 80 or older without prostate trouble. Therefore, it is not necessarily a disease of old age.

The natural or herbal healers contend that if the prostate engorgement can be softened and reduced in size, back to the normal proportions, then the flow of urine will once again be free and regular. On the other hand, some of my informants among the healers -- especially medical men -- also maintain that it is unlikely that the prostate, once it has flared up, can ever be brought back to its regular size.

From my consultations with pathologists I have learned that autopsies reveal that most men have enlarged prostates at any age above 40.

The prostate, once it is brought under control, can be kept under control only by following a strict regimen of eating, drinking, living and sane sex practices. You are definitely warned that such small or apparently inconsequential things as getting a chill, drinking a bottle or two of cold beer or a couple of cups of tea or coffee or a cocktail, eating a food that contains a lot of salt or having a prolonged sexual bout can cause a flare-up of the old trouble. Copious intake of fluids of any kind, especially alcoholic, prior to retiring is fraught with danger.

Indulging in the above practices will once again start the merry-go-round of hunting for relief and the use of the same methods and treatments that brought you relief before. But one of these days, if you keep this up, the methods that brought relief before will fail to work and then you'll be in real trouble.

So I urge you, if you have managed to bring your prostate condition under control and back to something resembling normal functioning, change your living, eating, drinking and sex habits to conform to those recommended by the hygienic ways of living. Then, and then only, can you be free from the danger of recurrence of your prostatic condition.

PELVIC STRUCTURES

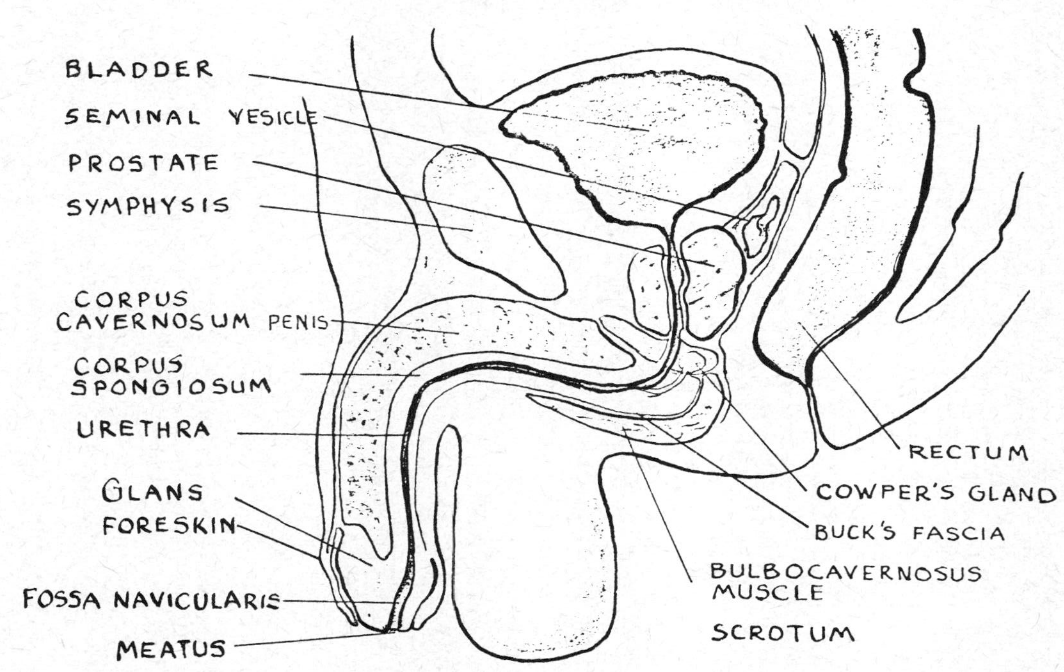

Chapter Fourteen

HOLD EVERYTHING!
IT MAY NOT BE YOUR PROSTATE!

If you begin to show signs of having problems or troubles with your genito-urinary system, you will, I'm sure, consult a healer of some sort and of course most men who are troubled go to a medical practitioner. Nevertheless, whichever type of healing you seek to follow, the first thing will be to tell your story to your healer and he will make an examination of some sort. Usually the first one, of course, is to feel your prostate by means of the rectal route, as mentioned elsewhere in this book.

There is no doubt in my mind that if you're past 40 or especially if you're past 50, even before you've said "Jack Robinson" your condition will be assumed to be a prostate condition -- usually prostatic hypertrophy. And if it is a medical doctor that you've consulted, it is a safe bet that he will undertake no treatment but will advise you to see a urologist or he will make the appointment for you.

Now I'm not suggesting that this is all done so casually, but I still maintain that by and large this is precisely what happens.

I also know that any good practitioner will put you through a series of tests to establish that it is a prostate condition before anything else is done. But again I suggest that in about 99 cases out of 100, when you complain of troubles in your genito-urinary tract, your complaint will be diagnosed as a prostate condition.

My studies, my searching and my personal questioning have convinced me that, without any shadow of doubt, not all of the troubles treated as prostate troubles are due to the prostate. It is my sincere belief that a great number of prostate glands are removed or enucleated that really do not require this type of treatment. However, I will concede that in practically every case the prostate was enlarged to a greater or lesser degree. Furthermore, I am familiar with many of the tests that are given to establish that it is a prostate condition from which you are suffering. Generally the medical profession will recommend seeing a urologist and the wind-up will be that the urologist in practically every case will recommend one of the four forms of prostate surgery.

I do not intend to go into the rhyme or reason why they do this and whether they are right or whether they are wrong but I do want to stress that not always when such situations arise is your prostate to blame. But the prostate, in my belief has become a real whipping-boy and whenever you show signs of trouble with your urinary system, your condition is immediately diagnosed as prostate trouble and you are treated accordingly.

If you went to a healer and complained of urinary problems, the first thing he would ask is if you get up at night and how often you urinate. Then he would ask if you have a strong stream or whether you have a nice arc in your urine and by your answers, he would judge whether or not you had prostate trouble.

It is my belief that any one of many conditions can look as though it were prostate trouble but really have little or nothing to do with your prostate. Here I'm going to suggest a whole big list of things that can go wrong and which can be diagnosed as prostate trouble whereas it is something entirely different: a stricture, a small meatus or external opening, a long adherent foreskin, enlarged seminal vesicles, infected seminal vesicles, impaired functional capacity of bladder, stone in bladder, pockets (deverticuli) in the bladder wall, tumor in the bladder, stone in ureter, kink in ureter, growth in ureter, kidney derangements (too many to mention); rectal disorders; hemorrhoids, polyps, fissures, cancer, inflammation, festula and others; nervous system; blood diseases; tumors, paralysis of the sphincter muscles, a polyp in the urethral orifice, growth or closure in the urethra, anemia, syphilis, diabetes or other glandular disturbances, trouble with the endocrine glands, distention of the bladder, excessive use of alcohol, side effects from various drugs, locomotor ataxia or general paralysis, inflammation of the fistula, or the effects of a heavy dose of monosodium glutamate in some food that you've eaten.

Now any one or many of the above ailments can create the condition known as dribbling and also make you get up two, three, four or five times during the night to urinate. Yet I stress, it may have nothing to do with your prostate.

Frequency of micturition is often brought about by cystitis, which is inflammation of the bladder.

Please remember that practically every male above the age of 40 has some enlargement of the prostate and, therefore, that alone does not mean that you have prostate trouble or that you have to have your prostate treated or that you have to have your prostate removed.

Let me cite a concrete example. If you, as many do, went out on a party or a drinking bout and then went to bed and slept like a drunken or drugged man for say, seven, eight or nine or ten or twelve hours, you would probably awaken with a badly distended bladder and then you would find difficulty urinating and probably your bladder might even become inflamed and various complications might set in.

This may lead you or even the practitioner to assume that you were having prostate trouble, whereas it was actually not the prostate's fault at all. However, in the process your prostate might have become enlarged.

Is salt an instigating factor in prostate trouble? But salt has been used for thousands of years and mankind -- even primitive man -- has used salt since time immemorial. True, but salt a hundred years ago or salt as used in non-progressive countries is not our purely chemical refined salt.

I would suggest that the man who is a heavy user of salt is much more likely to have trouble with his kidneys, bladder and prostate than the man who uses little or no salt, and even at the risk of being labelled a something or other, I can best illustrate my point by quoting from my book "Salt and Your Health":

"Like other purified minerals, salt has a tendency to raise the osmotic pressure of the body and to interfere with the passage of colloids through the membrane lining of the blood vessels. The tissues are adapted to a specific osmotic pressure at all times. Any matter which tends to raise this pressure above normal is attracted to the kidneys. The kidneys in turn eliminate the matter through a process which physiologists term 'selective excretion'. Large amounts of salt which are part of the matter raising osmotic pressure are drawn to the kidneys for elimination. As the kidney tissue itself appears to be sensitive to salt, it is understandable that time and a constant heavy intake of salt should cause it to undergo some damage. Even in the early stages, heavy salt use may inhibit the normal excretion of water by the kidney cells. In the later stages, Bright's disease is a frequent development. Some members of the healing professions recognize that salt is a significant factor in producing the ailment. Thus they often recommend a salt-free diet for such afflicted patients.

"Eventually, the persistent use of large quantities of salt also causes frequent urination in which only small quantities of water are voided at a time. It has not yet been proven whether such urination is caused by a partial paralysis of the blood vessels surrounding the organs or by irritation. However, either cause is invariably triggered by the heavy protracted intake of salt.

"Another result of high salt intake is affected kidneys in which poisonous and excessive sodium collects and causes a serious saturation. As a consequence, many sensitive, delicate tissues are damaged and their constitution changed. Finally this can and does, in my opinion, result in malignancy."

If you use large quantities of salt on your food -- that is, via the shaker route -- or even if you are fond of pickles, salt herring, olives, spiced foods, spiced meats and such (all of which contain large quantities of salt) you may have a condition that is created or aggravated by the salt in your food. This can cause irritation of your bladder, irritation of your urethra and various discomforts.

I have good reason to believe that the use of large quantities of salt in your food does positively contribute towards dribbling. It is my further belief that salt over a period of time causes a type of paralysis in your sphincter muscles and therefore urine will dribble out from time to time and it will be hard to control. Therefore, your valve doesn't shut off tight and often the bladder is slow to empty. This all happens because of the heavy consumption of salt in your food.

At the juncture where the urethra unites with the bladder there is a muscular valve that is known as and called the sphincter or sphincter muscles. These sphincter muscles act as a valve and they control the opening and closing of the urethra at this point, which thus controls the voiding of the urine. Evidently when there is a dribbling or a leakage it is due to poor control of these sphincter muscles.

Undoubtedly a paralysis of the sphincter muscles could bring about retention of the urine. It is a fact that paralysis of the sphincter muscles does occur but it is difficult to establish that it is a paralysis of the sphincter muscles that is causing the retention, and it could easily be blamed upon the prostate -- especially if the prostate were enlarged. As I have learned and mentioned previously, it is enlarged in most men. Well then, how could one distinguish between the paralysis of the sphincter and an enlarged prostate as being the cause of retention? I maintain that it is practically impossible to tell, and I am trying to establish a means of distinction or differentiation.

You can quickly establish whether or not I know whereof I speak by going on a strict diet for a week or ten days -- in which you will permit yourself no salt of any form, nor contained in or added to your food. At the end of a week or ten days you may be pleasantly surprised to learn that the dribbling and other discomforts in your genito-urinary tract have been greatly relieved or completely cleared up.

Then to this test, if you added the fact that you would take in no water or any other fruit or vegetable that contained a lot of water after four o'clock in the afternoon, you might learn that you don't have to get up at night to urinate or if you do, perhaps only once, and you may discover, as I said at the beginning of this chapter, it may not be your prostate at all.

Furthermore, I might suggest that chronic constipation and piles contribute towards making you think that you have a prostate condition ... or they might actually contribute to a prostate condition. Therefore, if you found a way to prevent constipation, this too might illustrate that it wasn't your prostate that was causing your trouble.

I might suggest that you use fairly good quantities of fresh prunes or figs or raw salads that will enable you to have normal bowel movements so that you will be bringing no pressure to bear upon your prostate.

Why not find out for yourself whether or not it is a prostate condition that is causing your trouble, by putting into effect some of these sensible, logical, simple methods that I advocate?

If to the above suggestions you would

add a good brisk walk of at least a mile or two a day -- preferably five miles -- or some fairly active physical work, it might help alleviate the condition even more rapidly.

Chapter Fifteen

ABSTINENCE AND HOMOSEXUALITY

From my investigations among celibates -- including cloistered monks, priests, teaching brothers and those who have taken the vows -- it would appear as though they suffer less from prostate disorders than the general run of the population. However, aside from the viewpoint of the prostate, it must also be recognized that people leading a monastic existence do, as a rule, live longer than ordinary people.

Their comparative lesser degree of prostate troubles could be due to the following reasons: (a) Fewer sexual relations or complete abstinence. (b) Not being rushed or busily engaged or involved in too many activities, they would not be preoccupied and this would prevent them from delaying urination and therefore they would have little or no trouble with their bladders. (c) There would be much less danger of continued sexual stimulation or provocation. (d) Their diets, in my opinion, would probably be better balanced with a tendency to have more of their own grown, unprocessed food. (e) A goodly number of these monks, especially among some of the orders like Trappists, Benedictines and others, do regular hard physical labor.

There are in our society thousands, yes, hundreds of thousands and maybe more men who practise total abstinence ... that is, abstinence from sexual relations with women. The reasons are many and varied. (1) They may be homosexuals. (2) They may have had their sexual organs injured and then removed, due to an accident or because of an abnormality at birth. (3) There are those whose sexual organs never properly developed. (4) Then there are those who have had their sexual organs removed for other reasons, like the eunuchs of old. (5) And last but not least there are those who are born or become neuters or the "third sex," as they are sometimes called, for any of the above or other causes or reasons.

There have been many schools of thought which have sought to advocate the abstinence from sexual intercourse of any form because it wasted the vital energy within the male body. The followers of this philosophy or way of life are convinced of the evils of sexual indulgence and the harmful results of relationships between men and women. Now I'm not going to call these abstainers from sex relations fanatics, crack-pots or lunatics but it is generally agreed that anyone who does not agree with the accepted line of thinking is of course a nut, a faddist, or a degenerate. I'm not going to become involved in such arguments.

I know that there are hundreds of thousands of men who, though not priests or members of a monastic order, believe that because of religious observances they should abstain from carnally knowing a woman. Well, if you have read this book, you will know precisely my position and feeling on the subject.

Here I would like to mention an unusual thought that has occurred to me. Each and every one of us has learned through the years that a muscle, a talent or an organ that is not used loses its strength, its tone and its power. This holds true for the muscles of your fingers, your arms, your legs, your back, your eyes and even for your sense of smell. Therefore, it stands to reason that if these organs -- that is, the sexual organs -- are allowed to lie dormant, they will atrophy or dry up or, to say it in a term that is widely used, they will become rusty and eventually lose their ability to function at all.

The bodily organs and muscles are made to function from the soles of your feet to the top of your head and any organs or parts of your body that are not used and exercised will become useless or cause serious trouble. Therefore, by not using your sexual organs or by infrequent use of them, you can run into prostate troubles.

We know that the body will prepare -- that is, the sexual organs -- the naturally required fluids and if they are not utilized and ejected at regular intervals, stagnation will undoubtedly cause complications ...

whether it is the various prostatic fluids or the seminal fluids contained within the seminal vesicles.

For an example that illustrates my point I can cite a woman's breast. Shortly after conception takes place the various bodily organs whose functions are required, begin to take on new tone and appearance. The mammary glands grow in size and when the child is born, the mammary glands are ready to provide the vital fluid food for the infant. Then again, when the infant has grown into a child and no longer requires as much of the milk, the milk supply dwindles. Then when at last it is no longer required, the supply ceases. That is nature at work in her natural inimitable manner.

Do you recall the famous experiment with fish? Let me tell you.

An ordinary pair of fish were placed in a tank of water located in total darkness. Each subsequent generation of fish had smaller eyes than the previous generation, until the fish were born with but slits instead of eyes. Then when these eyeless fish were placed in a tank where there was light, the exact opposite took place. Each subsequent generation had larger or more noticeable slits until eventually their eyes were normal once more.

So there you have the story. An organ that is not used will eventually become useless and will not function properly or it may become troublesome ... and that goes for your prostate!

There's an interesting sidelight that

came to my attention while writing this book and that is, "Do homosexuals have prostate troubles?"

When I first posed that question I was not in a position to answer it. But by contacting various practitioners, including a consulting psychologist, a pathologist and a few urologists, I came up with the answer.

Homosexuals do have prostate troubles. In fact, my contacts informed me that the incidence among homosexuals was even higher than in normal males.

I also wrote to an organization known as the Mattachine Society to see if they could or would undertake to gather this information for me, but I did not receive an answer.

Chapter Sixteen

PERSONAL HISTORY

I have a sort of confession to make and while doing so I wish to specify that it is being made with great reluctance, because it brings to light personal aspects that I am loathe to make public ... but make it I will.

Early in 1963 I began to gather data and information and do some broad reading on the prostate with the definite intent of doing this book. I sent far and wide for material on the subject and I purchased any book that I could locate that dealt with the prostate in any degree. I sent for and received research data on the subject from all possible sources available to me. You will see from the bibliography at the end of this book that my digging into the topic was rather broad.

Another and a most understanding reason for trying to get information on the prostate was that I had found I was running into urinary difficulties from time to time myself. This dates back to 1950, which means approximately 15 years ago when I was in my early 40's. The difficulties at first were not very serious -- just things like getting up once or twice during the night. Sometimes after a heavy bout of drinking (occasionally liquor but more often coffee or tea) I had to get up three or four times during the night. This interfered with my sleep and was generally displeasing, to say the least.

On other occasions I found that I had to urinate frequently during the day and it became progressively worse until I was urinating sometimes every hour or so. Then as the situation progressed, on a few occasions when I got up at night I found that I couldn't urinate readily. Sometimes I would have to wait some minutes and even half an hour and longer before I could get the stream flowing.

The trouble could invariably be traced to over-indulgence ... but to the best of my knowledge, not of sexual activity (because I watched the reactions rather carefully) but of drinking either alcoholic beverages or tea or coffee. I found that too much fluid prior to retiring was my chief source of trouble. I also learned that various sorts of baked goods, like pies or cakes that contained one or many chemical mixtures, would bring on a bout of semi-retention. I checked this out very carefully and found that the homemade baked goods with no baking powder or baking soda or other chemical treatments caused no trouble. It appeared that the trouble was caused by something in the cakes or pies or biscuits, for when I ate fruit or rice pudding for dessert I did not run into this trouble.

After a few bouts of slowed-up or painful

urination I learned a technique that relieved the blockage. I found that if I moved my legs up and down in a sort of goose-step fashion for some minutes or if I got out and walked at a fairly good stiff pace, the trouble could be relieved and the flow of urine would begin.

It further came to my attention that some nights when I'd go to bed after drinking fairly copiously and being very tired and sleepy I would not arouse myself when the first urge presented itself but would put it off because I was very sleepy and warm and lazy. Eventually, when I began to feel some pain in the groin due to distention and forced myself to get up, urination was very difficult and painful. This, I thought, was because I had allowed my bladder to become distended and perhaps this caused it to lose its elasticity.

I have tried to trace back the number of occasions on which I had sporadic retention during the 15-year period that I mentioned above. I am reasonably sure that this disability occurred on not more than two occasions a year during the first years, but I did notice that the attacks became more frequent as the years went by. That is, in the early years I had it happen maybe once a year or less, then it began to happen twice a year, say, and in the latter years it happened perhaps three or four times during the year.

Mind you, it was never severe or complete retention and after a few minutes or an hour or so of maneuvers, as mentioned above, the flow began ... slowly at first, but increasing at subsequent attempts to urinate as the hours went by.

When I was in Rawalpindi my friend, Mahmud Butt, took my friends and me to dinner at the best restaurant in that city. There a sumptuous meal was served to us. I recall the hot, tasty, light, crispy rolls that were placed before us. I went overboard -- they tasted so much like home-baked -- and I ate half a dozen. They were small and so light and oh, so tasty! That night I had trouble with my urine.

When I was in Hong Kong in the fall of 1963 I attended a farewell party for one of my friends who was leaving us and going to Alaska. We went to a fancy restaurant and enjoyed what is known as Peking duck. We had lots of soya sauce in our food which made us all thirsty. Then I must have drunk 25 cups of Chinese tea. These cups were not the conventional size but a small Chinese cup without a handle. Actually it is only about 1/2 or 1/3 the size of our normal American cup. But I consumed what would have amounted to 7 or 8 normal American size cups of tea.

That night I ran into serious retention difficulty. About four or five o'clock in the morning I had to get up and start walking the streets. Eventually the urine began to dribble, but very slowly. It took me all of the next day and part of the following day before the trouble eased up enough for me to resume my normal activities. This was unquestionably the most serious bout I'd ever had up to this point.

One of the first positive clues that I had

concerning fancy baked goods came to me when I realized that many or most of my urinary troubles took place on Monday nights or in the wee hours of Tuesday morning. Now I am a member of our local Lions Club and our meetings are held every first and third Monday. The meetings are the usual service club dinner meetings and our caterer invariably prepares an attractive dessert -- chiefly pie. The food was always well prepared and zestful, and I usually drank tea but occasionally I would take coffee. Then, as I mentioned earlier and am repeating, after many urinary bouts and some thinking I realized that most of my troubles occurred on Monday nights after the dinner meetings. When I missed a meeting the trouble did not occur. Then I began to abstain from the dessert and found I had no noticeable trouble. I soon learned that when I ate baked goods I had troubles and when I abstained I was free.

The reason that I am giving you this bit of personal history is to acquaint you with what I believe to be positive causative factors as well as the methods that worked for me to overcome the resulting difficulty. I learned that as long as I did not drink too much of anything and ate wholesome, decent, proper foods -- that is, mostly fruits and vegetables -- I had no trouble. My flow was normal, there were no complications, there was no pain -- things were under control. It was only when I went overboard that I ran into trouble. In those days, I admit, I did this more or less frequently. As you well know, partying, regular drinking bouts and over-eating on the wrong foods make up an important part of our civilized way of life.

I prefer to omit any detailed description of the pain and the aches and the burning and the horrible searing sensation that I felt in trying to get the flow of urine to start. Any man who has gone through it will understand distinctly and clearly how I felt... and as for the uninitiated, well, a detailed description of the predicament would be wasted.

I will enumerate here what I believe to be -- at least, in my case -- the direct or immediate causes of these bouts of total or partial retention of the urine:

1. Alcohol.
2. Liquids of any kind in copious quantities before retiring -- especially tea and coffee.
3. Baked goods containing baking powder or baking soda or other chemicals -- that is, pies, cakes, doughnuts, muffins, buns and rolls. I am especially suspicious of ready-mix and oven-ready kinds.
4. Foods that contain excessive salt and doses of other preservative chemicals ... olives, pickles, anchovies, salted peanuts, salt herring, kippers and processed and cooked meats.

The above are the foods and beverages that were the basic or traceable causes of my troubles with my urine. I will not definitely affirm that it was the prostate or that the prostate had anything whatsoever to do with it ... but these drinks and foods were, without any shadow of doubt, tied in with my urinary difficulties.

I cannot leave this part of my story without emphasizing that I regard bakery products of any and all kinds an important causative factor in urine retention. I do not know which one of the many chemicals used in the baking process is to blame but I feel that within that orbit of our food lies the root of most urinary or prostate disorders.

It must be admitted that the medical and other healing professions' opinions seemed unanimous in fixing the cause of urine retention directly and unmistakably upon an enlarged prostate, without taking into consideration the contributing causes that I have enumerated above. I state boldly that other factors are somehow involved that have little or nothing to do with the prostate, except that it is an ever-present organ that somehow gets involved. If the enlarged prostate was the guilty organ, then why did the urine eventually come through? Surely the prostate swelling or enlargement did not subside that quickly! How could it? I was undoubtedly aggravating it by my straining and repeated attempts to get the flow started. No, I am certain that the trouble is not always the prostate.

Now from the point of view of biology or anatomy, it might have been my prostate that caused all this trouble but when I avoided all of the things I just mentioned I had no trouble. I could urinate without any difficulty. So, therefore, I cannot see that I must attach the fault or the blame to a badly functioning prostate.

I realize that my thesis may be in direct contradiction to accepted medical and other healers' opinions, but nevertheless, I relate the truth in the most direct manner of which I am capable. I strive seriously to place the blame where the blame belongs. It was because I drank too much, usually tea or coffee, especially before retiring. It was because I ate baked goods, such as cakes, pies and prepared fancy rolls. It was because I was too lazy or sleepy to get up when I had the call. I repeat and emphasize that those are the things that eventually brought on the bout of urine retention. All or some of these actions might have affected or caused the prostate gland to jump out of gear ... or was it some other gland or organ? Nobody seems to know or care. Certainly no one is doing any work, study or research on the matter. I cannot connect sexual relations with these bouts but I do admit that while all these things were occurring I did partake in regular sexual relations.

Here and now I wish to boldly state, even at the risk of being repetitious, that I am not in favor of surgery for the prostate as long as any other rational sensible avenues are left open. But I just as strongly want to impress upon you the fact that if and when there is no other way, then surgery is the answer. It is safe, it is direct and in the hands of a good surgeon, a man who has your interests at heart, you can come out of the operation in better condition than you've been in for many years.

I say to avoid surgery wherever rationally possible. But when the chips are down and you require it and can find no other way, do not fear it. After you have had the surgery, you will probably be as good as you ever were.

When the surgery has been successfully completed, I beg you not to go on and continue with your health-impairing way of life. Change your diet and drinking habits. Avoid the excesses of the things that brought about your trouble and you will avoid other complications in the future, such as cancer of the prostate or other genito-urinary organs. Right here and now I want to tell you that these troubles will come back again even though you have had surgery unless you change your living habits. This fact has been clearly established from my investigations with people who have had surgery and went on drinking and eating as they did before. Play it safe! Even though you have had surgery, give up those harmful disease or cancer causing habits.

Chapter Seventeen

THE PROSTATE AND SENILITY

I have been unable to locate any positive figures relating to senility -- that is, as to whether or not senility is on the increase or decrease among those politely referred to as senior citizens. However, from my inquiries and personal observations, it is evident that senility is a vital issue and concern among folk who are getting on in years or, let us say, who have reached their three score and ten and beyond.

Is there any connection between senility and loss of libido? Senility, as a rule, affects only older people and it is conceded that as we grow older our libido decreases until it slowly ebbs away. Therefore I would suggest that there might be a direct link between waning sexual virility and senility.

Then there is a provocative question that I would like to ask, "Can one be sexually vigorous and senile at the same time?"

Strange but I have never encountered any reference or connection involving virility and senility in all my wide investigations and reading. I am, however, of the strong opinion that they are incompatible.

Now I go one step further and I claim that senility is the end result of the loss of sexual virility. In other words, impotency and senility run hand in hand.

Lest you imagine that I am referring only to the male members of the species in this instance, I want it clearly understood that in this chapter I am dealing with both sexes because senility does not appear to respect the sex of the individual.

While it is conceded that a senile woman might be brought to the point where she would indulge passively in sexual relations, this only indicates that she might be following the command of a stronger will.

For a man the situation is entirely different. He cannot be passive and have an erection. Thus coitus for a senile male is, in my opinion, impossible. Thus, my conclusion ... senility and virility are incompatible.

It is my thought that even when a man is what they call "over the hill" sexually, because of his varied interests in life, he may retain contacts, hobbies and interests that might prevent or slow down the process of senility.

It must be granted that a man who is sexually virile will be interested in and attentive to his female partner. By the same accepted logic, it is recognized that when he becomes impotent and has lost his sexual drive and desire he will no longer be interested in or be attentive to his mate and thus will no longer caress, make love to and fuss over her. Under such circumstances the importance of the woman's position in the household declines and she becomes more and more unappreciated and neglected. If the male, through the years, had been a potent man -- that is, sexually -- and a loving husband, in all probabilities he was attentive and flattering, thus raising the woman's ego. When this great stimulus is removed from a woman's life, drastic changes may or, as I prefer to believe, do occur.

It is established that prostate surgery does in many cases result in sexual impotency as well as sterility -- thus bringing to an abrupt end the sexual libido in many males. This is the case frequently among those who are at or about the three score and ten period. Well, as I mentioned above, because of a man's sustained activities and hobbies, the senility process for him may be slowed down ... but let's look at the wife's side of it.

When her man -- in many cases of true love, her one and only man -- has ceased to be attentive and loving, her big motivating force is allowed to starve for lack of attention. With the loss of her husband's sexual potency, her lifeline to her home and surroundings has been severed. This is especially true among devoted couples who have not found the need for a wide circle of friends because of their deep love for each other. When his attentions cease, it is in such cases usually too late and there is scant opportunity to find another male who might be attentive ... even if she were to desire and seek one. Thus, because of her husband's prostate surgery, she becomes senile ... slowly or rapidly.

Please believe me, this is not as ridiculous as it sounds. I am trying to suggest that prostate surgery, with the lessening or ending of the male virility, can be a direct contributing factor to the senility of women. In fact, I contend that it is a positive cause of female senility.

Among the medical fraternity it is generally accepted that senile dementia or cerebral arteriosclerosis occurs in middle aged or elderly patients without cause. I oppose this acceptance for I maintain that in all things there is cause and effect.

I have a most logical motive for writing this chapter. The reason is also a vital one because my investigations have revealed what might be a means of aiding women who are senile in recovering and regaining their normal balance. But even better still, this chapter may contribute something towards preventing senility in those who will read and benefit from the experience cited herein.

Therefore, now I would like to cite a case history and this case history is a strikingly important one for many reasons, one of the chief reasons being that this case history is that of a doctor -- a qualified M.D. with other degrees as well -- with over 50 years of active practice and wide experience. I am omitting his name and any other links to his identity. I ask you to read this section very carefully. Here are excerpts of his letters to me ...

"I was glad to hear from you. We are both in better health than last year. I have no angina at all, and my wife's mentality has improved greatly. As you doubtless remember I consulted all the BIG men in --------- and none gave me any hope but that she would get worse. I even took her to a famous clinic in Florida for three weeks in April '64. The doctor put her on hormone treatment with no result. I therefore used my own ideas. I gave her 1200 i.u. Vit. E. a day and 100 mb. B15 t.l.d. (pangamatin). Also since the first of the year I have given her three doses of Dr. Koch's Synthetic Survival Reagent.

"Re prostatism, I have been through the mill and know what it is like. When I began to have trouble to urinate in 1956, I thought I would be smart and have an operation before I had complete obstruction and damaged my kidneys. I went to a surgeon who had done a lot of surgery for me over the years, including prostatectomies, with good success. I went in one day and had my operation next day without being loaded up with antibiotics. The result was that I had a massive infection of the prostatic bed with a complicating bilateral orchitis. He then wanted to castrate me, which I refused. As soon as I got out of the hospital I took a dose of SSR which cleared up the infection but which left me with a great deal of scar tissue and atrophied testicles. I was in a worse fix than before with a very small stream, in fact little more than drops.

I finally had complete obstruction, and Dr. B-------- in S---------- was unable to put a catheter in me. He took me to the hospital. They also could not put a catheter in, so they drove a large trocar directly into the bladder from in front. After loading me up with antibiotics Dr. M--------- gave me a choice of bringing the ureters out on each side and wearing a rubber bag for the rest of my life; or having a plastic operation, to cut away the scar tissue at the neck of the bladder and take a flap from the anterior bladder wall, making a tube out of it and giving me a new urethra. He was very frank and told me that he was not sure that I could survive such a long operation; also he could not guarantee that the graft would take, in which case I would end up with the first operation. I chose the plastic operation, because I did not relish the idea of wearing a stinking bag for the rest of my life.

"It has been quite successful because I am dry and can hold my urine from four to six hours. Of course I am impotent ever since.

"I know of no cure for enlarged prostate. It seems to be a part of old age because bulls and dogs have it also. The only preventative that I know of is for a young man to go out and get a good dose of gonorrhea with a complicating prostatitis. This causes the prostate to shrink permanently, and does not interfere with his sexual life. There are drawbacks to this procedure, which are strictures in the urethra, which can be stretched up periodically or even excised surgically. Another great danger is that a man may not wait until he is completely cured before getting married and so pass it on to his wife with resulting pelvic inflammation and sterility.

"I have wondered since my own trouble why the G.U. men do not shrink the prostate up with deep X-ray. The great objection to this is that there is too much money in it for the surgeons and that they do not want such a simple cure. This also is a stumbling block in the cure for cancer."

"Since you are writing a book on the prostate I think that you should make it perfectly clear that there are some unhappy results to the operation of prostatectomy. First of course is that a man will in the majority of cases be completely and permanently impotent. This should be made perfectly clear to the victim so that he will be prepared mentally to accept the consequences. I fear that this is seldom done.

"Secondly, the consequences to the wife. If she is an extrovert and has many outside interests, it may even be a relief to her to be free of her wifely duties. However, if she is an introvert and is completely wrapped up in her husband and lives for him alone, then, as happened with my wife, when her husband shows no further interest in her sexually she may deteriorate mentally, become prematurely mentally senile.

"We were both in our thirties when we married, but planned on having two or three children. The first pregnancy, about two years after marriage, resulted in a miscarriage. The second was a tubal pregnancy which ruptured and she almost bled to death internally. My wife was determined to have a baby. The third pregnancy went to term and I took her to The R--------- Hospital, to the chief of staff Dr. F-------- where I thought she would be safe. She was then 41 1/2 years old and it was our last chance to have a baby. Instead of doing a Caesarean operation, which would have given both mother and baby the best chance, he left her in labour for 60 hours and then applied forceps to an occiput posterior head and dragged it straight through with a resulting complete tear into the rectum. He could have rotated the head as I have done many times and delivered it in a normal occiput anterior position. The baby was so badly exhausted and bruised that it lived only one hour. It was a 9 lb. baby girl.

"When I was in the hospital for pneumonia last January I did some serious thinking and decided that probably my wife's mental health was partly my fault. Before my operation I used to go to my wife's bed frequently where after a session of kissing and caressing we would have intercourse. As we got older these occasions became less frequent, but I always noticed that however long it took me to achieve an orgasm, my wife never relaxed her efforts to give me complete and satisfactory results. I resolved that when I came home from the hospital that I would treat her psychologically as well as medically. I therefore have been going to her bed almost every night, hugging her and caressing her with my hands, her face, her neck, her breasts and her thighs. For a long time I got no response, but now instead of turning her back to me, she puts her arms and legs around me as of old. She is also neater about her person and does her hair up nice again. She has also bought three new dresses this summer. She is quite forgetful, but so am I. Her mental improvement is marked. I have finally convinced her that I still love her and find her physically and womanly attractive; that if I were able to do so I would have intercourse with her.

"A woman's attitude towards sex is different from that of a man. A man is satisfying his own desires. A woman seeks by love and tenderness to give her husband complete sexual satisfaction; she does not seem to care if she achieves a climax herself or not as long as her husband does.

"This may seem to you to be a silly letter, but it expresses some points that I have never seen in textbooks."

I had mental compunctions about publishing these two letters. However, after giving the matter deep, prolonged, intensive consideration, I felt that these documents were too vital, too human to be denied publication. It is further my belief that these letters could be of material help to many people -- perhaps hundreds or even thousands. Actually I considered the frankness of the data concerning his wife's senility one of the most tender, touching, penetrating documents I've ever read in my life. Moreover, I found that the advice contained in this doctor's treatment of his wife could be a lesson for all men everywhere and if followed, could be the means of extending happiness to thousands upon thousands of women and preventing or even alleviating senility.

You may also understand after reading these letters why I deemed it advisable to withhold my friend's name and connections, as well as any name or place that would divulge his identity.

Chapter Eighteen

ARE WIVES TO BLAME?

By all the rules of marriage, according to a male viewpoint, a man should be able to have sex -- that is, sexual relations -- whenever the thought or the idea penetrates his mind and he possesses the physical ability to consummate the act.

As a matter of fact, I submit that this is a thought that is in the mind of practically every single man before he is married. Now I may be wrong but I believe I am right! I know that in my youth I looked forward to my marriage with one thought uppermost in my mind ... that I could enjoy or indulge in sex whenever the desire possessed me. And at that time it was always!

Only the passing of time proved that this wasn't the way it worked. I soon learned that the culmination of my sexual desires or fulfilment depended entirely upon my wife's attitude or whim. It worked out this way... Whenever she felt like sex, I had sex. Whenever she didn't feel like it, I did without. Sometimes a bit of cajoling or petting or pleading would work wonders. But at other times my pleading, no matter how prolonged or how plaintive, fell entirely upon deaf ears. From my inquiries I have no reason to believe that things are any different with other couples.

Well, if the wife does not consent to have relations whenever the demand is made upon her by her husband, one of two things will result. Either he will become frustrated and wind up with a prostate condition much sooner than usual or he will seek other means or other women who will provide him with the sexual pleasures that he desires or that his body demands.

Usually when a man desires sex he has an erection ... and like a balloon, what goes up must come down. It is my opinion that the proper way to reduce an erection is by fulfilment ... that is, having and enjoying sexual relations.

My experience has been that an erection does not die easily -- especially when you are young. The fact that your partner refuses to co-operate doesn't spell the end to your erection. You can't explain to your penis that the wife is indisposed or that she is "mad" at you for something or that she wants to teach you a lesson or that she is just plain ornery. The erection still persists and seeks gratification. Thus, when it isn't gratified and this provocative situation happens frequently or occasionally, you're going to have trouble ... and I suggest it's going to be trouble with your prostate, apart from mental perturbances.

If your body requests or demands sexual

relations every day -- and there are many men who want it every day and can stand it every day -- and yet your wife sees fit to allow you to have intercourse only once or twice a week or even every other day, your body and especially your prostate gland will not be happy about the situation.

I also know that many a woman looks with distaste upon regular sex. She doesn't mind coming across once in a while or if and when the sex urge is upon her, but she feels it is not incumbent upon her to provide her body for a man whenever the whim strikes him.

Now I'm not going to argue the matter pro or con. A woman may have her rights and refusing her husband when she wants to may be one of them. But I still think that by not providing him or not being willing to co-operate with him, she can be one of the contributing factors to a serious prostate condition. Therefore, women, if you want a sexually virile husband, if you want a loving mate, if you want a man who will have his prostate and thus be able to enjoy sex with you for many long years, provide him with sexual intercourse whenever he desires it or whenever the mood is upon him. I think it is cheap health and life insurance.

Chapter Nineteen

SEX AND YOUR PROSTATE

Does anyone know how long the sex act should take? Does anyone know the duration period based upon physiological or psychological requirements? I suspect the duration would vary with the individuals and also with the time, the place, the circumstances and the mood of the partners. It is generally conceded that the more virile, or what are called the best men, learn to perform the act for periods ranging from half an hour to more than an hour. Some men have made a study of the subject and have learned how to prolong the act, yes, well beyond an hour.

Through the years I have read papers, books and treatises on the subject as well as studying eugenics, genetics or any volume that might help in explaining the various methods of continuing the act of coitus far beyond the normally accepted period.

It is claimed that most sensuous women prefer and choose a man who has perfected the art of coitus prolongatus and among the extramural sororities (I do not mean whores) men of such distinction are most popular and in demand.

I am not particularly interested in coitus prolongatus per se at the moment. I am only interested in its effect upon the body ... specifically in this instance on the prostate gland.

To prolong the sex act is basically a violation of the normal function of the human body -- frustration to say the least. Every time the body or nervous system is brought to a point harboring on the climax the motor is cut off. This stop-and-go business continues frequently or is repeated a dozen or more times in one bout.

If the same principle were followed in driving an automobile -- that is, cutting down your motor as soon as you reached, say 60 m.p.h. and then before the auto came to a complete standstill, cutting in again -- think what this would do to your motor. There is no doubt it would soon cause a serious breakdown.

Now accepting the fact that the human body is a much better built and finer piece of machinery, yet cutting in and out 10 or 20 times a day or every other day would ultimately cause complications, to say the least!

Remember, I am suggesting that neither the motor car nor the body were constructed for this bit of manipulation. Let's face the situation squarely. Nature concocted the sex act to further her needs and to make it functional she made it pleasurable and desirable -- but again remember, specifically for her purpose.

Coitus prolongatus distinctly perverts and often seeks to defeat nature's avowed intent.

Now if I am talking to people who have never attempted or practised coitus prolongatus, then my reasoning may fall upon deaf ears. But all those who have indulged or do indulge in coitus prolongatus will readily understand my reasoning.

Look at it this way ... All conditions leading to the sex act have been fulfilled -- it is in motion -- the prostate and its attending ducts, glands and organs are functioning in unison. Then, just as the climax is about reached and finis is to be written to the act (as nature intended) the process is abruptly brought to a standstill. Then in a few minutes the process is repeated ... and this goes on again and again.

Thus, as far as the organs are concerned, it is frustration after frustration. It is small wonder that the prostate becomes hypertrophied. To me it is a wonder it doesn't explode into a million fragments.

Please believe me, I am not trying to create a hypothetical monster. I am relating a common occurrence in the lives of many men. It does take place -- it is real!

At this point you may ask, "Then does hypertrophy of the prostate occur only among men who practise coitus prolongatus?"

Well, that I do not know and I am in no position to answer. I do suspect, however, that it is one factor -- perhaps a most important factor -- but not the only factor. I do suggest that anything that deviates from the norm in regards to the sexual and urinary organs can be a contributing cause in prostate disease.

Because no writer, scientist nor investigator has so far pinpointed a specific cause of prostate disorders, I am exploring all likely channels . . . and coitus prolongatus strikes me as being a leading suspect in this deep mystery.

My own experience with coitus prolongatus has been that I sometimes developed an ache in the region of the groin. I could not under any circumstances claim that this was to my benefit. To speak truthfully, I would suggest strongly that the feeling indicated that it was contrary to the desire or wishes of my body and should be discontinued.

Chapter Twenty

COITUS INTERRUPTUS

Now we come to coitus interruptus which is known to the laiety simply as 'pulling out'. When pressed to make a decision concerning the foremost single cause of disorders of the prostate, I have, after due and profound deliberation, laid the blame directly upon the practice of coitus interruptus ... although because of the mechanics involved, I have listed it second, after 'withholding urination'. Coitus interruptus is jocularly referred to as a railway man's stunt ... 'pulling out on time'.

This form of sexual intercourse is practised in order to avoid pregnancy and the ejaculation, instead of taking place in the vagina, occurs in some prepared medium outside. How the practising of this unnatural act affects the prostate is not apparent or generally known but no one can deny that this action, at least during the early stages, does give a rather severe shock to the nervous system. I know, speaking for myself, clearly and to the point and without false shame or modesty, that at the moment of ejaculation I want to embrace and clutch my female partner to my heart with all the strength within me and smother her with kisses. But if you practise coitus interruptus, this delightful performance is not possible and you are not doing justice to your partner. Besides you may be causing serious damage to your nervous system, your prostate and I don't know how many other organs or glands.

I recall an incident that goes back more than 35 years ... when I was first married. I was told the story of a man who suffered a serious nervous disorder which was causing him to become a physical wreck. After making the rounds of the physicians of the city, no one could be found who could lay down the reason or offer or suggest a cure for his condition. However, eventually fate led him to a very wise and experienced physician who, after close consultation and investigation, asked him how he prevented conception during his sexual relations. The man reluctantly revealed that he practised coitus interruptus or the method of withdrawal.

The doctor then suggested that he practise normal sexual relations without the use of any apparatus to prevent conception ... no, not even the rubber or French safe. He asked him to try it for a period and then let him know how it worked out.

When the man returned for his next visit to his physician, his condition had improved to such an extent that it left little doubt that the withdrawal method of sexual practice had caused the trouble. Needless to say the individual did not go back to the practice of coitus interruptus and he remained healthy.

When I began the writing of this book on the prostate, I had completely forgotten the incident ... but when the term 'coitus interruptus' turned up, the story came vividly to mind. Through the years I definitely learned that coitus interruptus was certainly not a healthful practice. Rather, I had best say, and to put it a little more succinctly, I knew it was a harmful practice. Yet I and millions of other males or most other males do practise it ... perhaps with the exception of the peoples of India, China and other Oriental countries. Perhaps herein lies the reason why American or Westernized males have prostate trouble whereas those who do not live what we know as a modern life are free of it. This factor is well worthy of close consideration.

Now let us go through the motions of the practice of coitus interruptus ... and I want you to follow me closely, spiritually or bodily or whatever way you want, because this is important. Let us say that we are observers and we are watching a young male -- a youth -- practising coitus with his loved one. This is prior to the marriage state or might we call it illicit intercourse.

After the normal period of love-making, cooing, billing and caressing, the youth proposes sex and pleads to be permitted to gain entrance to his heart's delight. The maiden refuses and after much persuasion she gives the reason that she is fearful of the consequences of becoming pregnant. He then assures her that he will protect her by withdrawing prior to ejaculation. At last she consents and then the act is begun.

By then the prostate has prepared the young man for entrance by permitting the flow of the preparatory fluid. The sex act is then practised and enjoyed for let us say ten or fifteen minutes, which is a long period for an inexperienced young couple. Then as the young maiden feels her lover's pulsation, like a scared rabbit she swings aside or, true to his promise, the young man suddenly withdraws. There we have the young male panting, puffing in a hyper-state of excitement, and as the ejaculation begins he behaves exactly like an epileptic in grotesque convulsive ejaculatory throes.

Here I am describing precisely what I know to be true in my own case and in others through the years that I have been permitted to observe. To me a young man in this state looks exactly like a fish out of water. Normally he might be the handsomest, the most composed, complacent, wholesome looking young person in the world but under the spell of coitus interruptus he looks like a maniac or an idiot ... like someone suspended in mid-air, going through violent, jerking, spasmodic, frightening motions.

Now let's look at the other picture ... a young swain and his beloved who for any one of many reasons do not fear the price of illicit sexual relations. At the time when the ejaculation begins the couple are locked in each other's arms in a firm fond embrace, clutching each other in a paroxysm, welded into one being for those few moments. The firmness of the embrace prevents the convulsive movements. There is a chime, there is harmony, it is a confluence of body, mind and soul to the highest degree.

Please, now I ask you to picture the two scenes and then you may gather and understand why I say that coitus interruptus is first and foremost the one greatest single cause of prostate disorders.

Evidently the prostate gland must absorb this tremendous mental and physical upheaval. The prostate is akin to a shock absorber. But how much shock can even a shock absorber take? Through the months, the years, the decades of abuse, the shock absorber can no longer take the terrific hammering to which it is subjected and the enlargement or hypertrophy occurs.

I challenge any normal male, with the exception of celibates or those who have never had intercourse or who practise abstinence, to speak up and say that my delineation of this occurrence is erroneous or false or misunderstood.

Let me deal with one further aspect. In the lives of most men who have raised families there were times when the wife became pregnant. From the time that you decide to have the offspring or from the time that pregnancy occurred, by accident or design, there came into existence a complete freedom of sexual conduct. There was no need to practise coitus interruptus. Do you recall the pleasure, the joy, the exultation, the happiness that ensued? Well, if you don't, I do ... and I enjoyed and lived it up practically through the entire period of gestation. I recall these events and they were probably the happiest days of my entire married life and I looked forward to each night's session with longing anticipation. I say honestly, great were my expectations and greater were my fulfillments. Perhaps you may think I am making something of nothing but only one who has not felt these great joys would say that. Anyone who has felt them knows that they were every bit as true as I have described them.

In this present day and age men can avoid this harmful and I say debilitating practice of coitus interruptus by a variety of means as follows: (a) permitting his wife or partner to become pregnant, (b) using a French safe or condom, which I do not consider any great improvement, (c) vaginal douches, (d) the plastic ring or inter-uterine contraceptive, (e) oral contraceptives, which I warn against.

In practically every instance where you practise coitus interruptus you are paving the way for future prostate disorders as well as possible malfunctions of your nervous system. I further suggest that you are also contributing to possible future varied illnesses and diseases for your wife. I don't know which is the lesser or the greater evil or blessing -- I am not the one to judge. However the fact does remain that the practice of coitus interruptus can be avoided.

Without doubt the best way to eliminate coitus interruptus is by having children as nature intended ... but I am not running your life and probably at the age that most men will be when reading this book, that is not a vital consideration anyway. Therefore this chapter can be of great value to young men -- men who are about to be married or men who are just married. I say this to the women ... if you want to prevent your husband from having prostate trouble in the future, do not compel him to practise coitus interruptus. And young men ... if you don't want to run into prostate trouble when you reach the age of 40 or 50 or 60 then avoid this most harmful practice.

Have you ever heard of the term 'onanism'? Well, my interpretation is that onanism and coitus interruptus are one and the same thing ... that is, wherein the seed is wasted. This practice is harshly condemned in the Bible. If you will refer to Genesis, Chapter XXXVIII:9, you will see that it was considered a vile, vicious practice in those days and the Lord slew Onan for this practice ... and this goes back about 4,000 years or more. And who can deny that it is a vile, vicious practice today!

Now for a moment let us consider the use of condoms. At one time I felt that this apparatus did more harm to the female than to the male partner but I have had some change of heart on the subject. Closer studies seem to indicate that this synthetic means often tends to block or prevent normal ejaculation. During the act the violent, forceful back and forth movement tightens the covering around the glans of the penis, thus preventing normal ejaculation. You don't have to have a very vigorous imagination to quickly realize that this blockage, by preventing the forceful casting out of the semen, can have serious consequences, not only to the penis but to the urethra, the bladder and, of course, the prostate.

The present "Pepsi generation" is even making use of "saran wrap" as a contraceptive. In our modern civilized way we practise coitus interruptus, coitus prolongatus and other deviations, aberrations and corruptions that are not indulged in by any other species on earth. To me it has always been a wonder that more men and women did not wind up in the loony house, although I know that there are great numbers in such institutions now for no other reason than "sex."

Chapter Twenty-one

COITUS RESERVATUS

It is generally conceded and must be recognized that disorders of the prostate are invariably the result of disregard or abuse of the normal regular functions of the male. This is usually coupled with careless exercise of the sexual functions and above all, an end result of sexual stagnation.

I must warn against the practice of prolonged sexual excitement and stimulation without satisfactory termination, for this tends to congest the prostate. Of course this is a condition that is not generally encountered among older males ... it is the youth who compound this type of crime against the body.

Then of course there is the prolonging of the sexual relationship for extremely long periods without reaching an orgasm. This is also considered a vital cause of prostate disorders.

If you have ever indulged in a long bout of sex without gratification, you will no doubt have learned that the result is excruciating pain in the lumbar region of the lower back with penetrating pain and lead-like heaviness in the testicles and along the cords. Where there has been a continued or persistent erection for many minutes or even for an hour or two, the above condition invariably follows. The pain will even penetrate to the shaft of the penis and sometimes become excruciating and unbearable. In fact you can often feel this ache in the rectum and the perineum ... and when there is pain in this region, it is impossible to sit and even when standing, it is still severe.

My experience has indicated that this pain can be readily relieved by a sexual ejaculation.

While one is suffering from this condition, due to prolonging the sex act or sustaining an erection, he will eventually have to urinate and then the urination is painful and incomplete. This can lead to complete retention.

This condition can also result in changing the outward appearance of the individual. You can see the strained, drawn, haggard features of the afflicted. Upon encountering such an individual one can quickly see that he is suffering great pain. Sometimes he is unable to walk and if he can walk, his gait is slow and faltering.

We reach an impasse concerning the vital problem of sexual frequency. I call it a vital problem. It is a difficult, trying situation and after approximately 40 years of study of sex I am no closer to an answer than I was when I was a child. I frankly admit that I do not know what might be the normal frequency.

According to an old German rhyme supposedly written by Luther, twice weekly was the norm ... and here I quote it in German with the appropriate English translation:

"Zweimal zwe und fuenfzig sind hundert und vier.
Dies schadet weder mir noch dir."

"Twice fifty-two is a hundred and four.
This is a normal couple's score."

For some men seven times a week is inadequate. For others, twice a month is too much. I have known men and I have read of others, who require sex not only once a day but perhaps twice and even three times a day. This was not just on rare occasions but often for periods of days. It sounds incredible but if you will study the aberrations and abnormalities of sex, you will find that I speak the truth.

You will say that a man who is so incessant in his amorous proclivities lets his life's blood ebb away. This may be true and it may not be true ... but I do not concede that a man is physically weakened when his body demands and can indulge in sex any more than he is weakened by physical labor. I have yet to meet or know of the first man who suffered a stroke, a heart attack or other misfortune while indulging in sex. But it is also true, I must admit, that dead men tell no tales!

I wish I could say with any degree of certainty that sex should be indulged in twice a week, three times a week or every day ... but I can't and I challenge any man on earth to lay down a rule of sexual frequency and prove it.

There is a school of thought that maintains that it has never been proven that sexual intercourse ever added to the strength and well-being of a human being. They grant that it might create a feeling of well-being or peace of mind or physical satisfaction or it may flatter our ego so that we can thump our chests and say, "I am a man and this proves it!"

Whether they are right or wrong I am afraid that I cannot say with any degree of certainty. They are willing to go to the mat to prove their contention. And while it cannot be proven, to my knowledge, that sex ever improved the health of a man, they can show that it does materially affect or undermine the health of countless millions, and probably cite India and China as examples. Who is to gainsay these statements?

Here I would like to discuss with you another interesting, unusual and what I contend may be a dangerous sexual practice. You have no doubt heard about people who practise the sexual act and yet who do not desire to lose "the vital fluid" as they call it. These people maintain that the semen is a potent, vital fluid and should only be used for propagation of the species and as most of men's sexual activities are concerned with pleasure, therefore, they maintain that a great amount of this vital fluid is lost, causing serious, irreparable harm to the human male.

So they refer you to an art that authorities tell us has been practised by the yogis for hundreds of years and this art permits, according to their philosophy, greater satisfaction for both the male and the female yet does not allow the escape of the vital fluid. This act is referred to as "carrhiza." Evidently the reason behind this practice of carrhiza is to enable the male to conduct and practise sustained intercourse for many hours and with great frequency. This practice, it is claimed, allows sexual communion to be indulged in for periods of up to 8 or 10 hours at a stretch without fatigue on the part of either partner, but specifically the male ... without motion or effort and of course, without losing a drop of the semen. Furthermore, the only time that the fluid is lost or utilized is if they desire progeny. It is claimed that these yogis indulge in this method or art and they cite this as an example of how the voluntary muscles and glands can be controlled by the mind when the proper physical and mental development has been reached.

One John Humphrey Noyes, an American reformer who wrote a famous bulletin called "The Male Continence or Self-Control in Sexual Intercourse," was the founder of the Oneida Community and in his pamphlet he gave the complete details of his theory of 'Seminal Conservation'.

The famed Havelock Ellis, of psychology and eugenics fame, has stated that in his opinion this method of sexual relations is without harm to most men and may be of benefit to women because of the prolonged sexual contact which is preferable to 'coitus interruptus'.

It is claimed that this method was practised for more than 20 years by the participants in the Oneida Community without observable trouble or injury to the members.

In his written work Noyes clearly related his views as follows:

"This method of controlling propagation is natural, healthy, favorable to amativeness, and effectual. Only two children were born each year to the entire community and these were 'wanted babies'. The useless expenditure of semen continually is not natural. No animal wastes seminal fluid as man does. This is wasted energy and cannot be natural. Yet, it is equally manifest that the natural instinct of our nature demands frequent congress of the sexes, not for propagative, but for social and spiritual purposes. It results from these opposite indications, that simple congress of the sexes, without orgasm is the order of nature for the gratification of ordinary amative instincts; and that the act of propagation should be reserved for its legitimate occasion, when conception is intended."

I must admit that I am not in a position to judge the merits of the carrhiza or the method followed by the Oneida Community. However, I will not brush it aside and say that it has no merit. I consider the philosophies and the workings of the Community to be something beyond the framework of this volume. But nevertheless, I am very much concerned with the specific phase of carrhiza or coitus reservatus and the effect it might have on the genital and urinary organs, which of course, includes the prostate.

From the information I have been able to gather it would appear that the practice of 'coitus reservatus' tends to place a strain upon the genital organs, especially the prostate, to an even greater degree than does coitus prolongatus. Whether this does harm or creates other trouble I am not in a position to say and I don't know if anyone else is. On the other hand, it could be that an organ that is put to frequent or continual use grows stronger and probably enlarges. Then it is possible that this practice would cause it to harden, as would muscle, and whether the enlarged gland would cause blockage of the urine is something else that we do not know for I have never encountered anyone who has made a clinical study of this aspect.

You will note in the quotation from Noyes' actual words, "The useless expenditure of semen continually is not natural. No animal wastes seminal fluid as man does. This is wasted energy and cannot be natural." On the other hand, by the same token, does any animal extend the act beyond what we might consider normal? My observations of animals indicate definitely that the act is performed in the most forthright, direct and speedy manner to bring about an ejaculation and thus complete the act and the intended provision of nature. Therefore, I would say that the art of withholding the completion of the act is definitely unnatural. I will leave the problem with you for your further thought and consideration.

There are in our present day society a large number or proportion of men who seek to satisfy or who must satisfy sexually more than one woman. Even though the day of polygamy is gone and past, the fact that I have just mentioned, that a man is frequently called upon to satisfy more than one woman, is a part and parcel of our society. The art of coitus reservatus certainly looks like a logical solution to this problem but as to its benefits or harm, I make no attempt to evaluate this factor.

At times a man may be compelled to over-exert himself by the conventional method of sex indulgence. It may mean that upon occasions he may have to seek artificial means of arousing his passions or procuring an erection. Men will seek, on such occasions, and often resort to liquor and other potions which may be harmful types of food or drugs of a herbal nature or aphrodisiacs. Then there are instances where a man has a wife who is very passionate or she may even be a nymphomaniac. Under such circumstances, he is called upon to indulge in sexual intercourse more frequently than his body requires. Such enforced sexual arousement can be and I believe is a vital contributing factor in prostatic derangement.

A sustained high rate of sexual cohabitation, maintained over lengthy periods, by fair means or foul, can be a factor in prostatic hypertrophy. There may be further and even more serious complications and these practices may result ultimately in impotency.

Chapter Twenty-two

THE DANGER OF FORCING THE ORGASM

After three years of study and deliberation I have reached a conclusion concerning the major cause of prostate enlargement and I stress this fact and want you to take special note of it. Yes, I sincerely believe that I have found an important contributor towards prostate enlargement ... and this would occur just as easily in men of 40 as in men of 60 or older.

You see, every man seeks to retain his sexual prowess. Whether this is just the ego in a man or due to other factors, each and every man likes to feel that he is sexually virile. Well, there comes a time when, due to our mode of life, advancing age, our diet or some other reason, we are not as sexually active as we would like to be.

Now this especially holds true where one is married to a more or less passionate woman or one who enjoys sexual intercourse with comparative frequency. I'm not talking about once a month -- I'm talking about twice or three times or even more times during a week.

Well, as I mentioned above, when one combines too much drinking, too much high living, insufficient rest, wrong diet, long working hours and of course the toll of the years, one might not be as potent or as sexually virile as one would like to be. Thus, when the occasion arises and one engages in sexual intercourse, there is the desire to prove that one is still capable of an erection and of a proper orgasm.

If, as a mature man beyond middle age, you have never reached the state where you find it difficult to command an erection or reach an orgasm, then you are indeed fortunate. But many a man, especially beyond the age of 40, does occasionally run across the situation where an orgasm is difficult. So what does he do? He strains and strives and bends every effort to prove his manhood. And often by sheer willpower or by forcing himself, an orgasm is reached and he feels proud or content that he has proven his virility.

In my opinion this is a most important contributor to prostatic hypertrophy. If you practise or have practised this type of sexual manipulation, I warn you, I beg you, to stop immediately before you run into serious trouble. Sexual relations should be indulged in only when the body feels the desire for this act. Furthermore, the climax should be reached in a pleasant, natural manner. If it is reached in any other way, in all probabilities it will do more harm than good.

This causative factor has, to the best of my knowledge, never been mentioned or suggested by any other writer. I mention it because I think it is of vital importance and I believe that this practice should be avoided.

While masturbation is given as one of the leading causes of prostate trouble by many medical and other authorities, I would not entirely agree with that thesis. However, excessive masturbation is comparable in its effect and harm to the body to the forcing of an orgasm in sexual relations. That is, when a man -- either due to advancing age or the inability to normally perform the sexual act because of debility -- forces an orgasm, there is a similarity between this forced orgasm and excessive masturbation. In both cases the climax is reached due to "whipping" the body or specifically, the genital organs.

It is my sincere belief, from all the investigations and studies that I have made, that this forced ejaculation or orgasm is an important contributing factor in prostatic hypertrophy.

Chapter Twenty-three

THE LAST POST

After three years of gathering data, reading, studying and searching, I have reached the conclusion that the simplest means of handling a troublesome prostate is by surgery.

Now this statement, coming from a man who claims to be a naturalist and who believes in the natural way of doing things and who seeks to avoid medicine, drugs and surgery of any kind, is, to say the least, a complete turn-about-face. Perhaps I'll be called a hypocrite, a turn-coat, a Judas or even worse ... but I speak as I see the situation.

I have been asked, "If you do not believe in surgery, why do you recommend or suggest or advise surgical treatment of the prostate?"

Well, my experiences and observations have shown that in most cases when we become cognizant of a prostate condition or when we finally find out that it is the prostate that is the seat of the trouble, many years have elapsed ... and by then it is usually too late for the simple medical, herbal, naturopathic, manipulative and other non-surgical treatments. So you see, it is only because the condition is not quickly recognized or because we think it is something else that valuable time is wasted and thus, surgery becomes the only remaining avenue.

Besides, it is too much to expect a man who is 50, 60 or 70 years of age to change his eating and living habits. I think he would rather change his religion. Therefore I am facing the situation as it exists and not as I would like it to be. Realizing the frailties of human beings and knowing that not one man in 1,000 will follow a sensible, a proper or a correct way of living and diet, then I say that surgery is the easiest and the best means of dealing with a troublesome prostate.

The risk of death from surgery of the prostate is remote. It is practically non-existent today. The results aehieved by surgery of the prostate are most gratifying.

I sincerely believe that it is possible, if one will lead a carefully controlled existence, to avoid prostate surgery ... provided you have not reached the point of no return and you haven't had complete retention of the urine.

If you go to a surgeon with retention of the urine or other prostate symptoms, in practically every instance the surgeon will definitely not operate upon you until he puts you under his treatment and he will wait usually until the inflammation or the engorgement has subsided or at least, as he puts it, until the infection is under control.

Well, by this time you will probably be relieved of your troubles and if you had retention of the urine, you probably can urinate again ... either by means of a catheter or in the normal manner. Therefore, you can postpone the operation indefinitely or until you return to your old living habits and then you'll be right back again -- probably worse than before.

However, if you are intelligent enough and possess the strength of character to change your way of living and avoid the excesses and the abuses that have formed a part of your life until now, then there is some hope for you. Only by this stringent means is there a possibility that surgery can be avoided. Perhaps you have not reached the state or condition or point of no return.

You see, by having the prostate surgery, you are permitted to continue once again the selfsame bad habits or excesses that brought about the condition in the first place. So I lay the matter squarely before you and you are the one who must decide whether it will be the natural means of attempting to clear up your condition or whether you will accept surgery.

From my actual investigations, I learned that most men fear prostate surgery because if will lessen, harm, interfere with or remove, so they believe, their sexual desires or means of intercourse. Now here again, to my dismay, I must defend the surgical. My actual experience and investigations reveal that most men do not suffer any loss of sexual vigor by removal of the prostate ... or perhaps I had better say, the peeling of the capsule. Some of the men with whom I have conversed have stoutly insisted that they are better off sexually since their prostate surgery. It was their claim that the pain, the trouble, the inconvenience, the annoyance and the fear before had prevented them from enjoying sexual relations. But now that all of that is past, they are more inclined to participate in and enjoy sex than they have done for some years, or at least since they began to have prostate trouble.

It is admitted that in most cases the forceful ejaculation is no longer there. It may also be true that it may not be possible to impregnate a female. But apart from these two things, all other sexual factors remain normal or even improved.

Please believe me -- and I say this in all sincerity -- I have not been paid off by the surgeons or any other group or body to make the above pronouncements.

The adult prostate is in a continued state of activity and secretes amounts of 0.5 to 2 milligrams per day, depending upon the degree of androgenic stimulation. This secretion is voided with the urine.

The normal prostatic secretion as discharged upon ejaculation is a creamy fluid and is composed of cephalin, cholesterol, choline, citric acid, proteins, enzymes, electrolytes, comparable in concentration to that found in the blood plasma.

The pH of the prostatic ejaculate is about 6.6 which is close to neutral in the acid-alkaline scale. The pH of the semen is, as a rule, almost identical with the blood.

The fluids excreted by the prostate and seminal vesicles are believed to be instrumental in the maintenance and activation of the spermatozoa.

Acid phosphatase in high concentration is also contained in the prostatic secretion and this is continually present in the urine.

Upon ejaculation the seminal fluid rapidly dries and coagulates. Due to a most unusual procedure, after the lapse of 20 or 25 minutes, by means of a specific enzyme action, the coagulated semen remaining in the urethra spontaneously liquefies and is thus carried out by the urine. In cases where prostatic surgery has been performed this spontaneous liquefication does not occur because the impaired or removed prostate no longer secretes this de-coagulating agent.

After intercourse and the resulting climax, the seminal fluid remains almost entirely in the urethra -- because of the absence of the ejaculatory force to hurl it out. Furthermore, the seminal fluid hardening-dissolving agent is no longer secreted ... which means that the seminal fluid remains in the urethra and coagulates and forms a barrier, preventing the free flow of urine.

Thus, when a man who has had prostate surgery has intercourse at night, following which he goes to sleep, upon arising he may find difficulty or extreme pain upon attempting to urinate. To prevent this troublesome and painful incident from occurring, I advise you to always get up and pass urine shortly after coitus.

Chapter Twenty-four

SUMMARY

I have sought to trace back the history of prostate trouble or prostate disease but I have to admit that I could find few or practically no references that date back much more than a hundred years. Would this indicate that prostate troubles were unknown to our ancestors?

This I can hardly believe but I must admit that I can find neither reference nor methods of treatment of prostate disease in any of the older journals or books. There appears to be very little, if any, evidence of prostate trouble in medical history more than one hundred years ago.

It is, however, a fact that the word catheter was in use in the English language as far back as 1601. This would indicate that urinary, bladder or kidney troubles date back that far at least. However, as today the catheter in America is used primarily in prostate disorders, then they must have had prostate troubles at least 350 years ago. Of course, it could be that in those days they did not recognize it as being a condition that involved the prostate.

It is also of interest to note that the word "prostate" did not come into use until 1646. But let me also add that I have not come across the word "prostate" in any medical literature that dates back more than 100 years. Now I am not saying that it does not appear in any medical literature -- I am just asserting that in the hundreds of pamphlets, references and books through which I have searched, it did not appear. Evidently the medical profession has acquired the word but recently.

If you doubt my statement -- and I admit that it does sound hard to believe -- pick up a few medical books about one hundred years old and see if you can find any mention of prostate diseases. Does this indicate that prostate trouble is strictly a disease of modern civilization?

If coitus prolongatus and coitus interruptus are considered causative factors, then why would not history of prostate diseases appear in ancient or medieval history? I feel certain that coitus prolongatus has been practised by man for hundreds and thousands of years ... for sex is mankind's favorite pastime and thus man has always sought to prolong it to the fullest extent of his ability and experience. Then, as history reveals, there was no danger of a population explosion, there was lots of room in the world, and thus, there was no reason to practise coitus interruptus.

Maybe this form of sexual congress is a modern invention because in the olden days men and women didn't care whether or not they had two children or ten children. But today it is fashionable to have but one or two children. In fact, among many folks even one or two is too many. Therefore, it might be a fact that coitus interruptus is a prime offender and it is well worth careful study, thought and consideration.

About coitus reservatus I am not certain. You see, this practice is based upon the theory that expending the sexual fluid was weakening to man and this view is not shared by many. However, many sects have avoided or abstained from sex for this and other reasons.

One rather eminent authority suggested that benign hypertrophy was a married man's disease and this authority claims that few unmarried men fall heir to it. Well, my inquiries have revealed that single men and even celibates do get or are subject to benign hypertrophy, yet the incidence among unmarried men is definitely much lower than that of married men ... and that is also taking proportions into consideration.

There are no records to prove or establish whether or not sexually virile men live longer than abstainers or celibates. Yet upon checking the dates and years on tombstones, I am certain that cloistered monks and members of other indwelling religious orders do live longer than the average man in our civilized fashion.

My investigations reveal that most authorities recognize that one of the chief causes of prostatic congestion is brought about by long periods of sexual excitement before completion of the act. This is known as coitus prolongatus. It simply means, I presume, prolonging the act of coitus.

Now if along with coitus prolongatus the individual practises coitus interruptus, which means that the penis is quickly removed from the vagina before ejaculation takes place, actually interrupting the act, this, in my opinion, multiplies the risk of prostatic disturbance. Therefore, in combination, coitus prolongatus and coitus interruptus appear to be accessories to prostate conditions and are considered most undesirable and unhygienic practices. Both of these actions are biological violations which no other animal on earth knowingly or willingly practises.

Then, if the individual, besides the abuses mentioned above, adds the use of alcoholic beverages, as well as many cups of coffee and tea, and foods containing heavy doses of salt, then the offense becomes even graver.

Just what role, if any, do hot searing condiments and seasonings play in prostatic disorders? I'm referring to things like hot peppers, hot mustard, horseradish, black and white pepper and other pungent spices. Anyone who has had any experience with these caustic, burning condiments or seasonings knows that they do cause irritation and cramps in the stomach, as well as burning of the rectum. In fact, the burning sensation from these hot peppers is akin to having a red hot poker thrust into the anus. If you think this is a joke, ask anyone who has eaten these red hot peppers and seasonings.

In mustard, for example, there is a poisonous oil known as allyl isothiocyanate. This oil is absorbed from the stomach into the blood stream and it is claimed, with authority, that it damages every part of the body that it touches. Common sense indicates that the liquid into which it was made, and perhaps some of the volatile oils, before being eliminated has to pass through the kidneys, the bladder, the prostate and the urethra. Therefore, even this one specific item -- mustard -- can play a part as a causative factor in prostatic conditions.

I am sure that many readers of this volume will come up with the statement, "Shucks, man, it appears as though everything we do and everything we drink and everything we eat contributes to prostatic disorders. Well, how on earth can this trouble be avoided?"

My reply is, "Obviously this indicates clearly to all who will observe why derangement of the prostate is so widespread and why practically 90 out of every 100 males who reach 70 have had or do have trouble with their prostate."

Here let us pause and sum things up. To begin with I'd like to make the following positivations:

1. 50% of all men in America past 50 years of age have prostate trouble.
2. One-half of those 50% who have prostate trouble will sooner or later

wind up with or develop cancer of the prostate.

3. 50% of all males at or beyond the age of 70 years develop cancer of the prostate.
4. It is a safe bet that more than 25,000 cases of cancer of the prostate will be diagnosed in the United States during 1967. This definitely does not include undetected cases... that is, men who had prostate cancer but died of other causes.
5. It is estimated that more than 16,000 men will <u>die</u> of prostate cancer in 1967.
6. Prostate cancer ranks No. 2 among the cancer killers in America.
7. It is an absolute fact that more than 90% of all males in America can expect some prostate trouble during their adult life.
8. Getting up nights does not necessarily indicate prostate trouble. It can be due to the following cases: (a) too much intake of fluids; (b) irritants in drink or food; (c) harmful chemical additives in drink or food; (d) a consistent and heavy use of such things as condiments, salt and drugs; (e) stone or other obstruction in the urinal passage; (f) stricture of the urethra.

It is widely recognized that in America we have the highest peak of mechanization and industrialization of any nation in the world. And whatever statistics are available seem to suggest that we also have the highest rate of prostate trouble of any country in the world. The author postulates ... is there any connection? It also means that there is more leisure enjoyed by the people of America than any other country in the world.

It is a known fact that a man can violate practically every biological law and get away with it if he is engaged in an occupation that calls for hard physical labor. Farmers as a rule lead a life that entails consistent 7-days-a-week hard physical labor. Farmers have the lowest incidence of prostate disorders of any segment of the American population, too.

I'll leave this with you for your consideration!

Now all the measures obtained and suggested within the pages of this book may prove ineffectual if the condition has become too far advanced and catheterization may have to be resorted to ... but at least these suggested practices can do no harm. We are avoiding any action that might aggravate the condition and in most cases they will probably bring relief and a great deal of benefit.

Common advice often imparted to sufferers, by people seeking to be of help to one troubled with troublesome urination is to cut down the water intake ... believing that if one drinks less water, then one would need to urinate less frequently. This is basically true, but on the other hand it tends to make the urine strong and irritating which is definitely not in the patient's best interests.

Often when men have to get up two or three times a night they don't regard this as being too serious, because again they think it is caused by advancing age. At the present time I know a few people who, when they discuss the prostate and advancing years, say, "Well, I am having a little trouble but I'll wait another year or two and then get the darned thing taken out and I'll be all right again."

Now believe it or not, this is a most prevalent form of thinking among men in America. They seem to believe that it is inevitable and therefore they put up with the difficulty until they get up enough courage or run into serious trouble and then they have the prostate removed. I consider this a tragic state of affairs -- something akin to willful neglect and stupidity. But I don't know whether or not I can blame the individual because that is what he is generally taught to believe and thus it has become the broadly accepted practice.

Then, too, there is a notion about in some quarters that men also have something akin to a menopause and therefore many men regard this as being just one of the phases. I do not believe there is any justification or clinical proof for this assumption, yet you'd be surprised how widely accepted this fairy-tale has become.

If you already have had some signs of prostate troubles, then you had best be alert, take stock and be careful. Here are some suggestions that you might follow to your advantage.

Never go to bed with a belly full of water, beer, liquor, tea, coffee, juices or any kind of liquid whatsoever. Just remember, don't go to bed with your body saturated with fluid. If you follow no other simple principle, even this one point may save you one heck of a lot of trouble and perhaps a serious, painful and troublesome bout with retention of the urine.

For anyone who has had the slightest touch or warning of prostate trouble I suggest that he go light on citrus fruit of any kind, be it grapefruit, lime, lemon or orange. Yes, I am aware of the fact that citrus fruits are widely used and often recommended in prostate conditions but I am telling you emphatically ... anyone with any sign of prostate disorders should lay off the citrus fruits and citrus juices.

I would strongly advocate that you give up salt in any form because no matter where I have investigated I have found that salt is a contributing factor. You should try to eliminate the salt even from your cooked foods and never, ever use the shaker. Every morsel of salt that you put into your body (I mean sodium chloride) has to be excreted and it has to go through your kidneys and through the urethra and the prostate, which surrounds or forms a part of the urethra, and it definitely does irritate all of your genital organs, but especially the prostate gland which I believe hypertrophies because of sustained salt intake ... which means it is continually bathed and soaked in a saline solution.

It is wise to remember that you do not always excrete in the same day all the water you drink during that day. If you consume foods containing large amounts of salt, the water will be held in your body until it is salt-saturated and only then will your body excrete it.

I would strongly advise that you take at least three glasses of water daily. It would be better if you divided this intake to two glasses in the morning and one glass in the afternoon, rather than vice versa.

Whenever nature calls, empty your bladder promptly. It should not be necessary to empty your bladder oftener than once every two hours and if you stop drinking any form of liquid after four or five o'clock in the evening, there should be no call for you to get up during the night. However, one emptying at night is normal and is definitely no cause for concern.

It is my belief that long sitting bouts do aggravate or even contribute to prostate disorders. Therefore, walk or stand whenever possible -- don't sit for any great length of time, especially in those soft easy cuddly chairs.

Under no circumstances whatsoever should you force a bowel movement. Never ever strain. Let nature function in its own way and time.

Avoid all foods that contain baking powder or baking soda. Better still, avoid all baked goods.

You can do yourself a big favor by

avoiding all chemically processed foods; that is, foods that contain any chemical additives.

Eat natural, wholesome foods.

Avoid a heavy protein intake.

Then remember, too, that the food you eat today will seldom be excreted today. In fact, it takes anywhere from two to five days for food to be digested, metabolized and excreted. Also bear in mind that a lot of the water you drink does not come out as urine but is excreted with the faeces as well as in perspiration and tears. Therefore, you cannot excrete water that has been used elsewhere. It is best to remember that if you don't take the fluids into your body you won't have to get them out.

For your counsel, I want you to remember -- definitely -- you should never attempt to have sex on an erection that is created and sustained by urine. It is advisable to avoid prolonged sessions of sexual intercourse, but do not undergo long periods without sexual intercourse. Regular sexual relations are essential for the well-being of the human being. Sexual arousement without gratification can be harmful.

I have attempted in this volume to give the various treatments, practices, methods and therapies of the different healing professions. However, my investigations clearly reveal that even within any given profession the form of treatment may vary tremendously. Then, too, it is clear that certain treatments are popular and used by most of the different healers. For example, the hot sitz bath seems to be popular in practically all fields.

Some physicians recommend prostate massage and others definitely abstain from and frown upon any such treatment.

One medical authority -- in fact, a mighty high medical authority -- suggests that only a small percentage of people suffering from prostatic disorders "really need any surgery." He goes on to say that "the eager and radical surgeon will disagree with this statement" but many years of experience prove that the majority of men who have symptoms of prostatic disturbance causing bladder disturbance can be kept in comparative comfort for an indefinite number of years.

This same authority goes on to say, "Why the stress of conservatism? Because more than half the causes of true enlargement are associated with inflammation, so that the enlargement producing the obstruction to free urination can be greatly reduced by simple measures and surgery avoided. There is no doubt whatever that too many men are operated on unnecessarily for prostate gland enlargement."

In writing this book on the prostate I did not seek or attempt to decide which is the best method to heal or correct the condition once it is found to exist. With the exception that I am in favor of surgery in extreme or terminal cases. I want to emphatically declare that I am not in any way bound or beholden to any of the healing professions nor do I have any preferences or prejudices for one over the other. I want it clearly understood that my beliefs are those of a naturalist ... and I use the word 'naturalist' rather than that of naturopath. You see, I do not believe in any kind of healing. It is my belief that the human body alone can heal itself if given the opportunity. When I say the body must be given the opportunity, I mean exactly that ... not just playing at it. The transition must be complete and unfettered. However, to begin with, all causative factors must be removed.

I also recognize that all of the healing professions have their practitioners and adherents. I have nothing against them nor do I hold any brief for any of them. Each and every one of the arts serves its purpose. Granted, some of the professions demand lengthier studies and schooling than others but I do not set myself up as a judge as to which is the best form of healing. I do not think it is wise to assume that a medical doctor is more proficient at handling physical impairments than a medical herbalist or an osteopath or a chiropractor or a naturopath.

My experience has taught me that all of the healing professions have performed to the benefit of mankind. Therefore in this volume I am giving the various methods or treatments as followed by the various healing arts or professions. But I neither advise nor suggest one treatment or therapy over another. Furthermore, as I stated, I believe in the natural way and stress that nature, if given an opportunity and no obstacles are placed in the path, can correct practically all of the human ailments without the use of drugs, potions, pills, injections, manipulations, heat, color, electricity or whatever other ways and means the various healers have discovered and used.

It is my suggestion, however, that all of the methods be studied or at least read carefully and then a decision reached as to the mode and method that you would prefer to follow for alleviation of your problem.

Furthermore, I want it positively stressed and understood that I recommend no man's practice and no man's product. This clear and unmistakable statement is made not to avoid responsibility but merely to emphasize my position.

Giving advice is very easy and also it makes one seem so erudite, but I also caution that it is filled with grave risks. Most respected healers will permit themselves the privilege of giving advice only on rare and safe occasions. Therefore, I advise the layman to play it cautious, especially where the prostate is concerned.

I have spent more than three years studying, questioning, gathering data and engaging in wide correspondence in order to gain knowledge to write this book on the prostate. I have also lived through most of the situations, treatments and practices outlined in this book. After all this, I desire to stress that I am not a healer of any sort nor do I pretend to be one, nor would I want to be one. I am an investigator, a chronicler, a searcher and I prefer to accumulate the information and lay it before you and let you decide your own course of action.

No two prostatic situations are identical. Therefore, what is good for one is not necessarily the right thing for another. For this reason I advise the would-be counselor to keep silent and not pretend to be an authority. Let the sufferer seek advice from those who are most qualified to give advice. I suggest to anyone who is suffering to seek and find the most qualified man in his vicinity, be he an allopath, naturopath, hygienist, chiropractor, herbalist, osteopath, eclectic or any other ... but make sure that he knows his business!

YOUR PROSTATE

Its functions and malfunctions as well as all known methods of

TREATMENT AND PREVENTION

TWO VOLUMES IN ONE

-- o --

Volume Two

INTRODUCTION

This section is devoted entirely to means and methods of treatment to alleviate prostatic disorders. Herein I encompass the treatments from all of the healing arts and professions. I have contacted healers in all fields and have asked them for detailed information concerning their treatments for prostate disorders and retention of the urine. Furthermore, I have carefully studied in detail each and every one of the methods in this section of the book.

At this point I would like to emphasize that I do not now nor at any time advise self-treatment. I say this in all sincerity ... and not because I am afraid of offending the healing professions by suggesting otherwise. There are among us those who can follow instructions as outlined in self-treatment courses. There are also those who can find information that will enable them to treat themselves successfully. However, because there are so few who are capable of doing this, I strongly warn against self-treatment. It can be dangerous!

No doubt tens of thousands have treated themselves to their physical benefit. Through the years I have met and have been acquainted with many of them. But the main reason I caution people against self-treatment is because people are prone to make errors in judgment, or become careless, or lack sufficient knowledge. Then, too, there are many other reasons -- most of which centre around lack of experience. Under such circumstances and conditions, self-treatment can be harmful and even dangerous. People in general, but especially those who are ill, do better with sound leadership.

I believe better results can be obtained by placing yourself under the care of some established, accepted practitioner. He need not necessarily be a surgeon or a medical doctor because there are other accepted, reliable fields of healing -- naturopathic, osteopathic, chiropractic, homeopathic, herbalistic and others. But I do sincerely suggest that you consult some responsible experienced practitioner who can guide and help you.

I am not attempting to persuade you as to which one of the treatments offered you should take. Personally I do not approve of one over another because I have no proof that one is any better than another. The only thing I am sure of is, when your prostate disorder becomes severe enough and painful enough, due to procrastination, self-treatment or even misdirection, there is only one answer and that is to see a capable practitioner.

While there are many healers in different fields, who claim that prostate troubles of practically all sorts, including the most advanced and severe, can be cleared up or definitely improved without surgery, I am not convinced that this is true. From the knowledge that I have gained through studies and reading and discussion, it is my opinion that there are many cases of prostatic disease, especially those of long standing, that do not respond to any other treatment.

From my consultations with practitioners in all fields, I find that many of them admit that in the final analysis -- when all else has failed -- surgery is the only answer. Therefore, a capable urologist can be a prostate sufferer's last hold on life.

Chapter One

WATER TREATMENT

This is commonly referred to as the "sitz bath." It is believed that cold water tones up muscles whereas hot water relaxes them. When hot and cold water are used alternately it is claimed that they help in a natural way to stimulate the body tissues and organs.

The recommended means of operation is to sit in a tub of hot water for about 15 minutes or until the lower part of the body is heated up thoroughly. Then the hot water is drawn off and cold water put in its place. The patient then sits in this for 5 minutes.

There are different thoughts on this phase of the treatment. Some think that the change from hot to cold should be drastic. Others think that the change should be gradual. I, on a broad attitude, oppose the drastic method because of the effect that the severe temperature changes may have on the body. Again, that is precisely what some practitioners attempt to achieve, for they claim that under such circumstances drastic treatment is required or called for.

The depth of the water need only be sufficient to cover the umbilicus.

These hot and cold "sitz baths" are considered of pronounced value for releasing obstructions causing difficulty in urination.

Where one is unable to partake of umbilical immersion in the hot and cold sitz baths, due to any one of many circumstances, hot and cold towels or cloths can be utilized. The use of hot and cold towels is the simplest form of the "sitz bath" treatment. This treatment should be continued for approximately 1 1/2 hours ... the longer, the better, according to old practitioners. The towels should be applied over and under the lower groin, between the legs. Seek to cover as much of the genital organs area as possible.

The sitz bath and the hot and cold applications have been in vogue for centuries and were for many, many long years the only method of gaining relief from retention and prostatic difficulties. Therefore, even in this modern day and age, these techniques should not be laughed at or ignored.

When using the sitz bath, the temperature of the water should be as high as the body can stand it. The duration should be anywhere from 20 minutes to an hour. The accepted practice is 15 minutes hot and 5 minutes cold, repeated up to 3 times at one treatment. This procedure can be followed a few times during the day.

Chapter Two

HERBAL METHODS

Now we will deal with the herbal treatments of the prostate and under this heading we will give a variety of treatments.

Here is a treatment used by Dr. Ethel Wells. She found this a very effective herbal remedy for prostate troubles...

"Parsley Piert Herb
Elderflowers
Buchu leaves
Wild Carrot

Equal parts. Mix.

"Use 1/4 ounce of each to produce one ounce of the mixture. Add 1 pint cold water and bring to the boil. When water boils, remove and allow to cool. Drink half teacupful after meals, three times daily."

Another herbalist says: "An excellent medicine for enlargement and weakness of the prostate gland may be made by infusing equal parts of Fleabane, Hydrangea and Saw Palmetto berries, half an ounce of each, in a pint of boiling water. Allow to stand until cool. Strain. Dose: two to three teaspoonsful before meals, three times daily."

Here is another herbal treatment for

suppression of urine:

"Boil 3 tbsps. of watermelon seeds in one pint of water; strain and allow to cool and then take or administer a teaspoonful every hour till relief is obtained."

Prostate Gland (Inflammation of)

Causes - Usually caused by sexual excess, weakness of the muscles, impurities in the blood stream, taking of strong cathartics. Improper diet which causes a diseased liver, kidney and bladder, thereby causing inflammation of the prostate gland.

Symptoms - Pain and tenderness in the fork of thighs, painful urination.

Treatment - Diet is of first importance. Alcoholic liquids, tea, coffee, and the use of all stimulating foods and drinks are strictly forbidden. A person suffering from this disease must have a diet consisting mainly of fruits, vegetables and grains.

Constipation is nearly always present in this condition, and great benefit will be derived from the frequent use of hot enemas, as often as three times a day. A high enema as hot as can be borne of either catnip or valerian gives great relief when there is much pain.

A slippery elm poultice is extremely beneficial; apply between the legs, in the fork of the thighs.

Equal parts of gravel root, and clivers, or peach leaves, or either one used alone, using a teaspoon to a cup of boiling water. Drink one to four cups a day, more or less as needed.

For an injection in any bladder trouble,

take a teaspoon of golden seal, one-half teaspoon of myrrh, one-half teaspoon boric acid, pour on one quart of boiling water, and steep thirty minutes. Inject with a catheter, connecting the catheter to a nozzle of a fountain syringe and hang up high, so the water will flow freely. Everyone should learn to use a catheter. This solution is wonderful to heal bladder trouble, when the causes are removed. It is very powerful to destroy poisonous mucus or inflammation in the bladder.

Prostate Gland (Enlargement of)

Causes - Enlargement usually results if inflammation is not properly treated.

Symptoms - Hard lump is present in the fork of the thighs, or rectum, which becomes very painful when pressed. Difficult and painful urination.

Treatment - Follow the same treatment as for inflammation of the bladder.

A sitz-bath at temperature of 105° to 115° F. is excellent in relieving the enlargement when due to congestion. Remain in the sitz-bath from twenty minutes to an hour. The diet as given for inflammation of the prostate must be strictly adhered to. Massage is beneficial, also electrical vibrator.

Here is a list of herbs that are used to promote the flow of urine, referred to as diuretics: Broom, buchu, clivers, couch grass, hydrangea, juniper berries, pareira, parsley, parsley piert, pellitory, pipsissiwa, shepherd's purse, stone root, uva-ursi, wild carrot.

Chapter Three

OSTEOPATHIC METHODS

Here is a letter I received from a well known, successful, highly respected osteopath, in reply to my inquiry requesting treatment for a prostatic sufferer with urine retention. I will quote it ad verbatim:

"At your request I will try to answer your questions.

"If a patient presented himself with a bladder retention and was in great pain, I would of course catheterize him immediately to relieve the pain. If he were not in great pain, then I would examine him to determine the causative factors.

"If the prostate were enlarged and boggy, I would use a Bio-Cold Ray machine to treat the prostate through the rectum to decongest it. If this failed, then catheterization.

"If the prostate was enlarged, hard and nodular or rough I would catheterize at once and do blood chemistry, especially alkaline-phosphatase and sedimentation rate. This would help establish whether or not it were cancer.

"If I can keep the patient from having

too many catheterizations, I would use a prostatic exercise. I do not believe in using finger massage of the prostate as it increases fibrositis. You are familiar with the prostatic exercises as I taught you this in St. Catharines.

"I would also place the patient on a proper diet. Eliminate all milk and milk products except butter. Then have him use the following supplements: Super Eff, 3 capsules a day. Cytotrophic extract of Beef Prostate, 3 tablets a day. Vitamin A & C. The dosage would depend on a urine analysis. If albumin were positive and any casts present I would use one tablet every hour for several days and then 4 a day. Calcium Lactate, 3 tablets on arising.

"If the urine were alkaline, I would use apple cider vinegar, 2 teaspoons in a glass of water 4 times a day.

"There are many other possibilities but I don't have time to write about each one. Hope this will assist you on your project."

I found this exercise that my osteopathic friend demonstrated to me and had me practise, very good and most exhilarating and I could see and believe that it could be of help to prostate sufferers. So I am giving you the exercise as he described it to me and if you did this exercise in the morning and before retiring for about 10 or 15 minutes, it could give strength and tone to your innards. Most certainly this exercise could never do you any harm and I suspect that it might do you a great deal of good.

Lie down on your back, preferably on a

hard surface like the floor or a bench.

The first and most important part of the exercise is done by drawing the knees up to the chest and making sure the knees and ankles are kept tightly together. If one opens the knees when pulling them up towards the chest, it ruins the entire exercise.

Then spread the knees apart and bring the soles of the feet together. This is done while the knees are held as high as possible.

Next, kick the legs out straight so when they are straight the heels are two to three feet above the floor.

Then let feet drop to the floor.

Repeat this ten times morning and evening.

Another exercise suggested to me...

Lie down with ankles bound together by either a piece of rope or a strap, and try to pull them apart... but do not bend the knees. Then separate ankles by means of a block of padded wood and try to bring them together. Then do the same exercises but with the knees bound or separated instead of the ankles.

The principle of the exercise is to exercise the muscles of the hips -- normalizing the muscles of the pelvis. You will need the following simple equipment: (a) a piece of rope or a belt and buckle, long enough to fit around your ankles or knees and (b) a block of wood (2 x 4) 6 inches long and padded to eliminate sharp corners.

Now I suggest that you try the following exercise to improve your body tone and the functions of your organs.

Have a bar built or hung in your bedroom -- one that will allow you to reach or hop up and suspend yourself from your arms without your feet touching the floor. Then swing or jerk yourself so that your body will hang free and loose. This tends to align your inner organs, even including your spine. Allow yourself to hang by your arms, wiggling your body for a few moments or minutes as your strength allows. Do not exhaust yourself!

Here is another osteopathic treatment used by a well known successful practitioner, including case histories. I quote ad verbatim again:

"Mr. A. S. an elderly little bachelor, about 59 years of age, has been known to me as a 'guest' at my health rest home for several years. He used to come summertime for a week or two weeks vacation. On one of these vacations, he requested an examination in the office. During my examination, I discovered that Mr. A. S. was having an enlarged Prostate. He complained among other symptoms, of pressure in his lower back and also of difficulty in starting the flow when urinating.

"This is one of the early symptoms of cutting off the urinary channel, or urethra. The prostate gland is the shape and size of a chestnut, when it is normal. It is located in the interior of the body where it can be felt by digital examination, about three inches within the rectum. It surrounds the upper part of the urethra. When it becomes enlarged, its cells swell up at first; then they become hardened and sometimes to the size of a fist.

"About four years ago, Mr. A. S. was examined at my rest home when he was advised to take a month of intensive treatment, which would include fasting, short wave diathermy and special exercise. So-called 'massage of an enlarged prostate' which consists of rubbing it within the rectum is useless. Yet it is being done in the medical field. I prefer to teach my male patients to take the knee elbow position and drop on one shoulder or the other while in that position, in order to drain the pelvic structures. I recommend the same postural exercise for women because the uterus is the homologue of the prostate gland embryologically. Women develop enlarged wombs for the same reason that men develop enlarged prostates. It is estimated by medical authorities that every second woman has an enlarged uterus when she has reached the age of 50, or earlier. Every second man has an enlarged prostate at that age. The enlargement of this important pelvic organ can be prevented by postural exercises from adolescence and youth, onward.

"Mr. A. S. did not take advice four years ago. He went home and went about his business. Last June 17th he returned with a troubled state of mind. His physician who had been catheterizing him every morning and every evening, told him that he must have an operation for the removal of the tumorous prostate, because it was dangerously enlarged. Mr. A. S. arrived at my rest home about ten o'clock at night and he confessed then and there that he felt uncomfortably full of fluid. Since I believe in teaching my patients how to be independent of doctors, I forthwith proceeded to teach Mr. A. S. how to insert a urethral catheter in order to enjoy the thrill of being independent of somebody else in withdrawing fluid from the bladder. He really filled a quart size jar full of foul smelling stuff. The patient was relieved and wanted to kiss my hands for teaching him.

"The next morning the same performance was repeated and the following eight days, Mr. A. S. catheterized himself morning and evening under the guidance of his physician, my humble self. He was a desperate little man and didn't even believe that I would get him out of this mess, but he had given me 'the chance' because he did not want to have surgery, for removal of that organ.

"At the end of eight days, he began to pass 'water'. The man was so thrilled when he began to urinate freely, that he collected the stuff just to look at it and see how much he voided 'naturally'. He literally voided about three quarts per day from then on, because his diet consisted of diluted lemon juice, a glassful to the lemon, and diluted grapefruit juice, a pint of water to the grapefruit. He was given three glasses of liquid, three times daily, for the first two weeks. In the meantime, the laboratory findings improved. The first urine showed 'pus' cells. The blood picture showed an increased number of white blood cells, which is an indication of inflammation; the water and lemon and grapefruit juice diet, cured his inflamed prostate; in the first four weeks. Its size reduced considerably. In the first digital examination, the prostate could be palpated by inserting the finger about one inch. Its size, which was fistlike, could be felt by inserting the finger as far as it could go. At the end of the month, the prostate was about the size of a small tomato. Naturally, Mr. A. S. was thrilled because he was better. He even indicated his desire to continue his treatment at home, in order to save money. My recommendation to him was to remain here for ten weeks in order to clear up his condition and to build him up in his general health. The little man's occupation is one of a factory shipping clerk and he was advised to build up his health in order to be strong enough to endure his job and not to get a recurrence of pelvic congestion. He took my advice and had a wonderful summer. He is a small man, about 5'5" in height, and weighed at the beginning of his treatment 122 lbs. At the end of four weeks, his weight was 102 lbs. I had to remove 20 pounds of his bodily wastes in order to make him consume his excess weight from the prostate gland. At the end of 10 weeks, his weight was 138 lbs. He left a grateful patient. The case report was obviously dramatic! IN A PERIOD OF 10 WEEKS, A DISEASED PROSTATE WAS MADE OVER!"

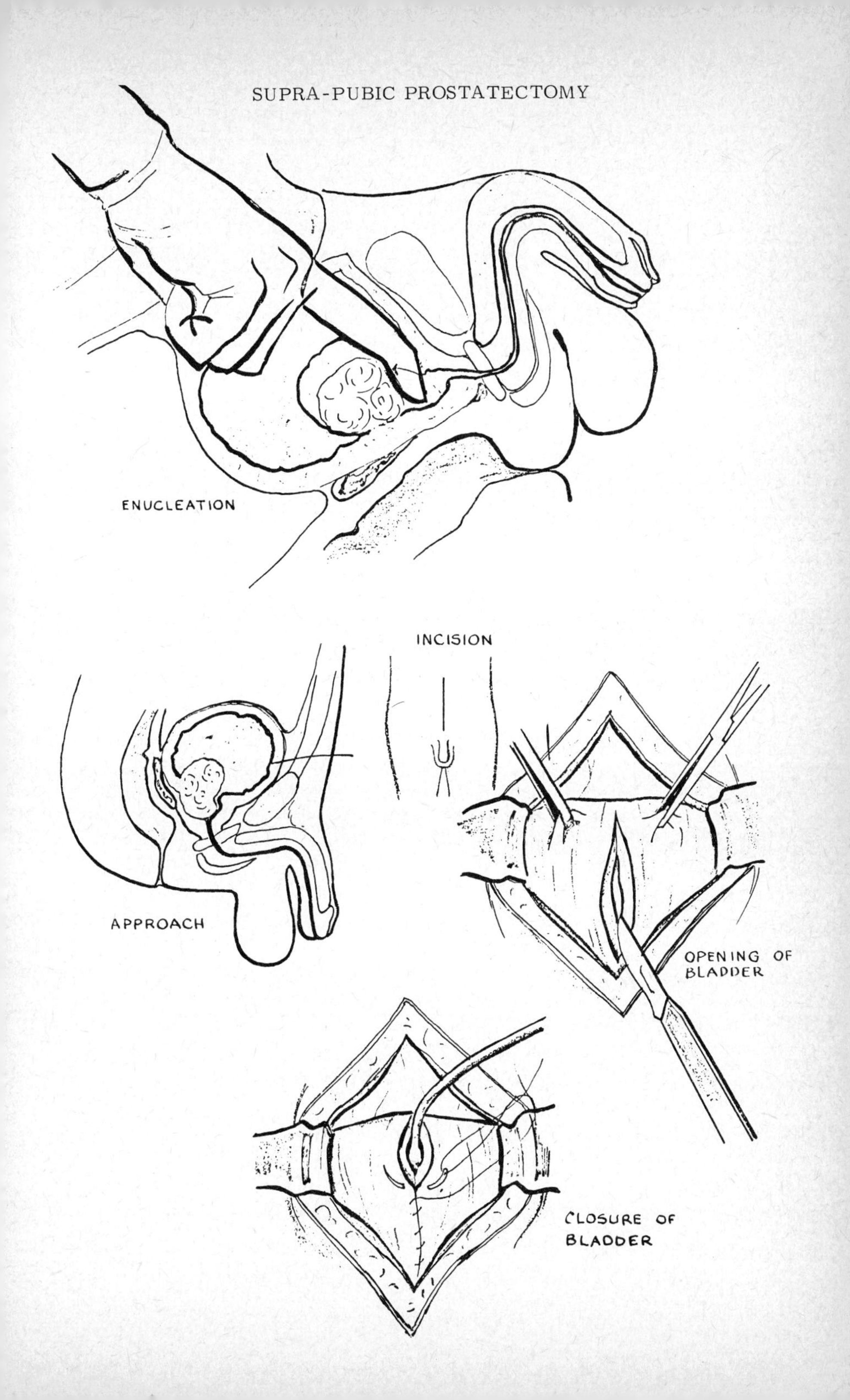
SUPRA-PUBIC PROSTATECTOMY
ENUCLEATION
INCISION
APPROACH
OPENING OF
BLADDER
CLOSURE OF
BLADDER

Chapter Four

SURGICAL METHODS

It is expected and understandable that when all other means of treatment have failed the last resort is surgery. Unfortunately this is not the wisest course because often when at last a recalcitrant patient consents to undergo surgery his physical condition might have deteriorated to such a degree that the chances of success from surgery are rather slim.

Now this may sound drastic or hopeless and you may say, "Well, if I'll need a surgeon eventually, why not a surgeon at the start?"

Well, it's like having an injury to an eye. You try to treat it by the simplest means possible and only when the situation becomes difficult or endangers life does one resort to surgery.

Under such circumstances many surgeons demand a week or a month or even longer for the patient to be built up or to recuperate before undergoing the knife. Yet it is often true that in some cases this is not possible because of serious complications that have arisen and surgery must be risked lest the patient succumb.

Modern techniques, however, have a means of clearing up situations that will then permit surgery without any grave danger. Surgeons are reluctant to take patients where the risk is great and most of the good surgeons will absolutely refuse to operate where the chances of success are narrow.

There is, however, another side to this story. Often surgeons remove prostates and patients undergo surgery where other methods might have succeeded. I am convinced that a goodly number of prostates are removed or enucleated that could have been saved and healed by other means of treatment.

It is no joke -- let's put it that way -- for a man to lose his prostate unnecessarily ... especially if he is a young or middle aged man, say a man under 60. No matter what is said pro and con, there is a danger of becoming completely sexually impotent and also, in practically every case the ejaculatory ducts or the means of ejaculation are interfered with or entirely impaired. Furthermore, the various forms of surgery often impair or remove other glands and vessels. Therefore it is not advisable at the first sign of prostate trouble to resort to surgery and have your prostate removed. However, it is estimated by good authorities that 70% of men sexually potent prior to prostatectomy retain their virility after the surgery.

It has been my experience that most

practitioners in any of the healing professions will do their very best to clear up a prostate condition according to their own methods of healing. When the situation involving the patient's health deteriorates beyond their control, they will of course recommend a urologist or surgeon. Therefore, it is my belief that the patient would be well advised to consult a capable practitioner and rely upon his good judgment. My inquiries for the past few years have revealed that most medical doctors will promptly refer you to a urologist when you come to them with prostate troubles. It is, of course, simple logic to understand that once he recommends the urologist, the chances of surgery have greatly increased. In fact, my inquiries also reveal that once you are placed in the hands of a urologist or surgeon, the chances are at least ten to one that you'll have one of the various forms of prostate surgery.

My position is neither for nor against. I do recommend, of course, that you use every possible method to clear up your trouble without resorting to surgery.

Now we will deal with the various types or kinds of surgery . . .

Today as this volume is written, urologists have at their disposal four alternate courses or types of effective surgical procedures to follow in dealing with the prostate and these methods are followed in cases where there is no malignancy.

If must be clearly understood that no single operative approach is applicable to all cases. Certain cases and certain situations demand certain specific types of surgery. Thus the best of the urological surgeons practice in perfecting the techniques in all four operative measures used in prostate surgery. When they have mastered these four techniques, they are then in a position to render the best possible service in the interests of their patients.

Trans-urethral Resection

This method is also referred to as the closed method of surgery, where no incision is made in the exterior body wall. The surgeon penetrates through the urinary passage by means of a resectoscope. This is a tiny hollow tube-like instrument that is fitted with a magnifying telescope and a light which enables him to see what he is doing. On the inner part of the tube a movable loop has been placed. This is made of hair-like tungsten or platinum wire. When all is in position a high-frequency current is permitted to pass through the loop. This incises through the tissues and cuts and cauterizes at the same time -- thus cutting down bleeding to a minimum. Then the surgeon removes the lacerated pieces with the selfsame instrument.

My studies reveal that two types of trans-urethral prostatectomy are used regularly. One is by means of a platinum loop through which a high-frequency current is used to cut tissue. In the second method, a tubular steel knife is utilized... and this method is referred to as the "cold punch." The first method is referred to as the

TRANSURETHRAL PROSTATECTOMY (Resection)

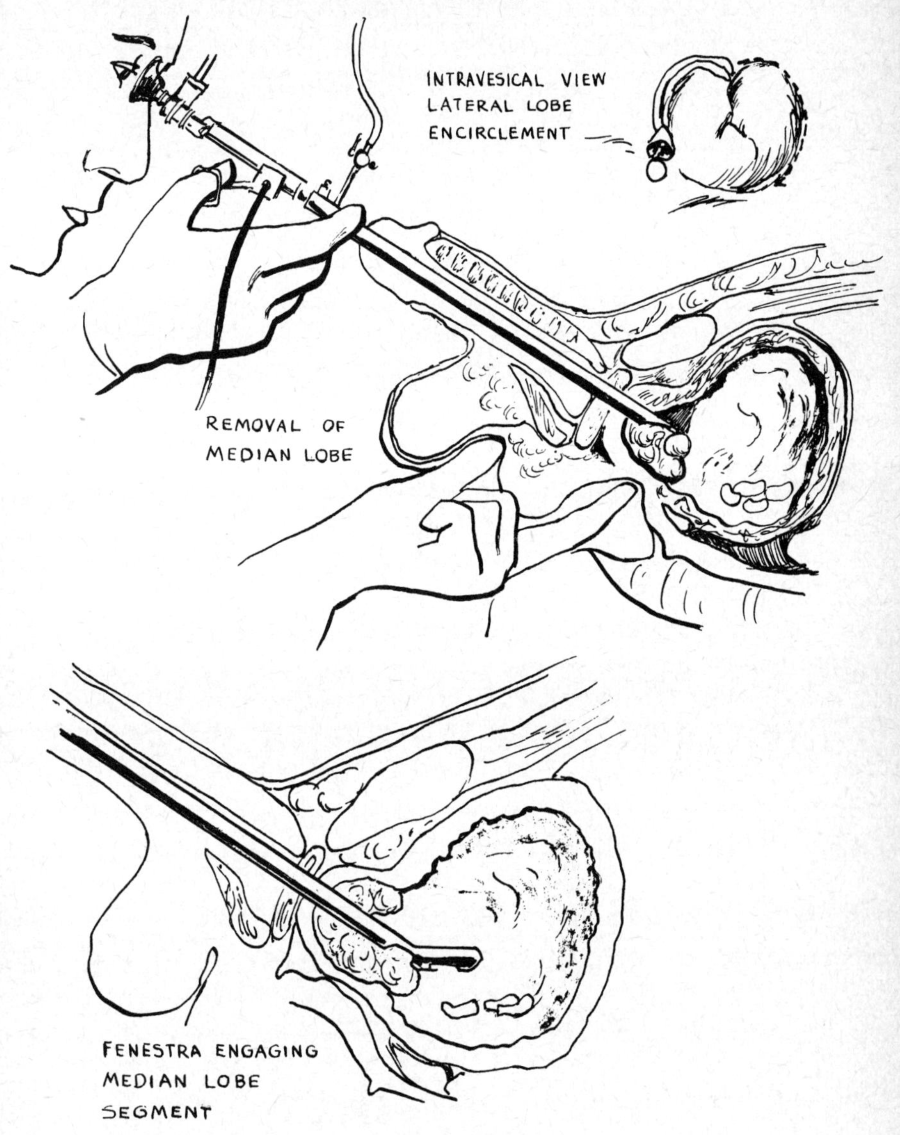

COLD PUNCH TECHNIQUE
WITH TUBULAR KNIFE

trans-urethral electroscopic method.

In both methods a tube is inserted into the penis through the urethra and the tissue is cut away and allowed to fall into the bladder and then it is removed piece by piece.

Those who use the "cold punch" method claim that healing is much quicker because of the absence of charred tissue which results from the use of the high-frequency platinum loop.

It is admitted that this trans-urethral method sounds most complicated but this form of closed operation involves little or no danger and the patient is ready to get about again in a few short days. He is even voiding urine without the use of a catheter in from three to five days and is back at his home in something like a week.

It has been my impression, judging from conversations with many people who have had this form of surgery, that this is the least satisfactory of all four methods ... inasmuch as the surgeon does not have the complete control that he can exercise by his three other means. I further believe, and urge the reader to bear in mind, that the chance of recurrence of prostate trouble is greatest through this means of surgery.

It must be remembered that each surgeon has his specialty and he will prefer his specialty and the operation that he does best which is only natural. Yet what that specific surgeon does best is not always in the best interests of the patient. But who is there to gainsay or dictate to a surgeon the type or means of operation that he should follow?

I have learned that some surgeons think that the trans-urethral prostatic resection involves some dangers that are not found in the other methods of surgery ... in spite of the fact that it is the simplest and affords the least danger to the life of the patient. Actually a trans-urethral resection demands greater experience and judgment than any one of the other three operative methods. I must also mention that this form of surgery is preferred by most patients who have been erroneously or otherwise led to believe that this is the simplest and the best and of course the least confining.

Frankly, I warn against pressuring the surgeon for any one form of surgery. Either you trust your surgeon or you don't. If you don't, then don't go to him. If you do, let him work on your prostate in the manner he thinks and believes best. Then again, you can inform yourself by study and inquiry ... or it may be in your best interests to talk it over with a good internal medicine man (a diagnostic specialist) and then decide on the type of surgery to follow.

One very good surgeon -- a man of high repute -- told me that he likes to get inside and see and feel what he is doing. Then and then only can he do justice to his skill and to the patient's welfare. From my studies and discussions with other surgeons, I must agree with this man.

It must be stressed that where there is a large or a massive gland to be concerned with, trans-urethral resection is definitely not applicable.

Supra-pubic Prostatectomy

This is the type of surgery most widely practised throughout the world for prostate removal or enucleation ... and it can be performed by any capable, proficient surgeon without special training in urology. In days gone by this was considered a most dangerous operation but improved techniques have made it probably the least dangerous and the most effective of the four methods known. Records indicate that inasmuch as risks in lives are concerned, all methods are about the same. There is very little risk and a very low, low rate of mortality in any prostatectomy irrespective of method.

It is definitely established that the end results by means of supra-pubic prostatectomy are better than by all other means. This form of surgery is ideally adapted for extra large glands which close examination through a cystoscope have revealed to protrude upwards into the bladder.

In this method an incision is made in the abdominal wall and the bladder is exposed. Then the bladder is opened and this makes the prostate gland available for the work at hand. The technique followed here is to peel out or enucleate the gland from its capsule.

This method appears to allow for the cleanest and neatest removal or enucleation of the gland. There is less danger of hemorrhaging and other complications by this method of surgery. It is shown by experience that if no complications set in, the patient, by means of the one-stage supra-pubic operation, can be completely healed and urinating in 10 days to two weeks.

This operation used to be done in two parts -- that is, allowing the cut in the bladder to heal before completely closing the incision. Now it is all done by means of one operation.

This method does have its disadvantages. It is definitely not applicable where there is cancer involved and where the patients are in poor health or obese. Because it is trans-abdominal and cuts through the abdomen and the bladder, bleeding is often difficult to control.

The surgeon cuts through the abdominal wall and then through the bladder and then with his forefinger he reaches into the urethra and breaks through the mucosa. Then he peels away the ball of prostate tissue. This is referred to as enucleation, for the prostate capsule is usually left intact.

When the adenoma is removed from within the prostate capsule, the bleeding is usually controlled by means of the insertion of a Foley bag catheter.

While this method may require a longer stay at the hospital, because of the slower healing involved, it is, in my sincere opinion, by far the best and simplest of the four surgical procedures.

All surgical prostatectomies require regular irrigation through an indwelling catheter and irrigation is usually given every hour for some days, and in some cases every half hour and again in other cases of a

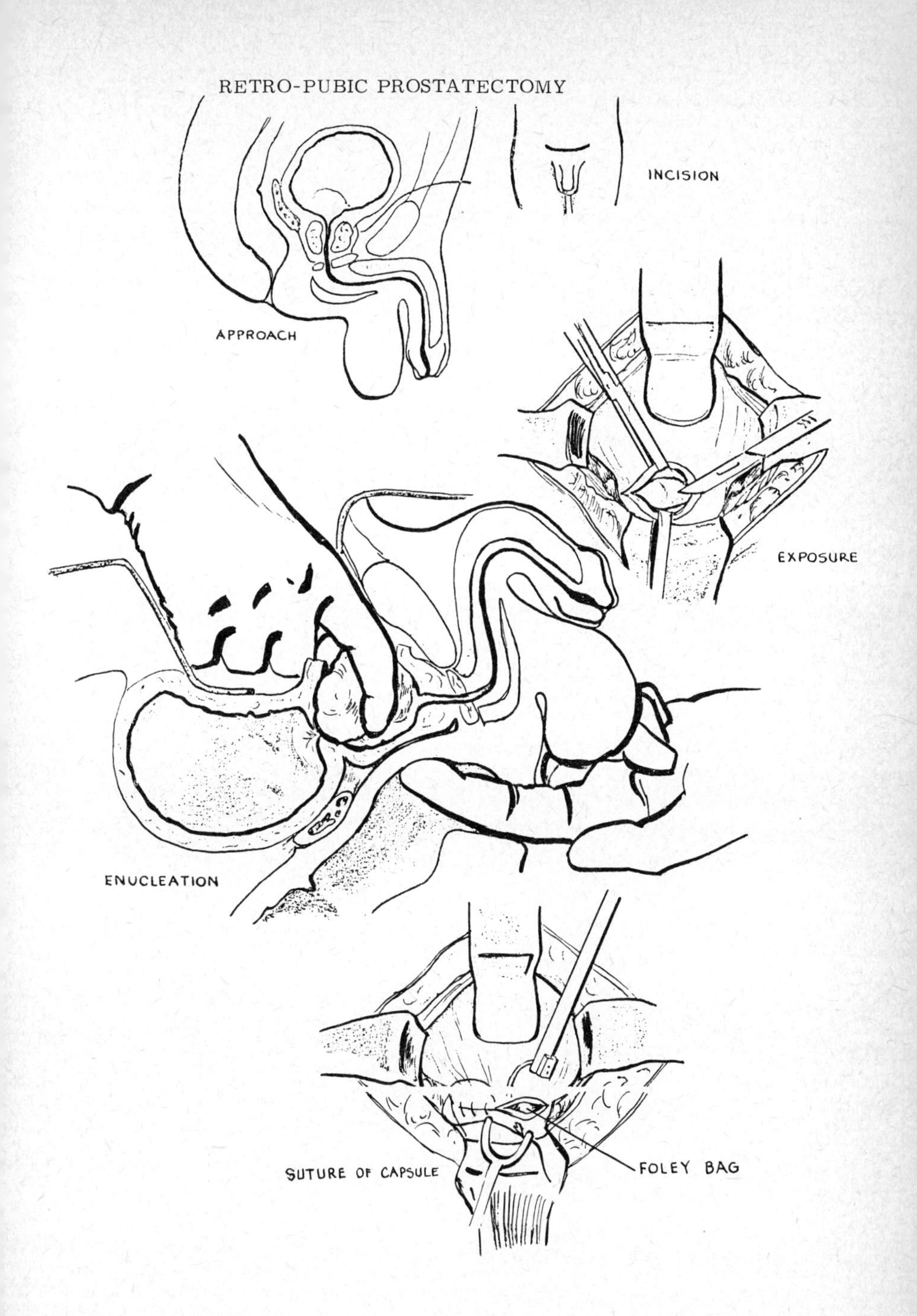
RETRO-PUBIC PROSTATECTOMY
INCISION
APPROACH
EXPOSURE
ENUCLEATION
SUTURE OF CAPSULE
FOLEY BAG

more serious nature, every fifteen minutes. This is to prevent obstructions caused by coagulated blood or other residues.

Retro-pubic Prostatectomy

This method of surgery was developed within the past fifteen years and is but a variation of the supra-pubic approach. Where the prostate is of exceptionally large size and situated high in the pelvis, the retro-pubic approach is ideally suited.

The retro-pubic method is not advised or applicable in cases where tumors or stones of the bladder exist ... or where the median lobe of the prostate is exceptionally large. It is definitely not recommended for prostate cancer.

It is definitely recognized that the retro-pubic approach is technically a more difficult procedure than the simpler supra-pubic method, as it requires more retraction and a deeper wound.

The general approach is similar to the supra-pubic operation but instead of entering the bladder as is the case in the supra-pubic, the anterior surface of the prostate is exposed. The prostate is enucleated in a similar manner to that of the supra-pubic method except it is not done through the bladder.

The one big advantage of the retro-pubic over the supra-pubic is that the bladder cavity is by-passed and not entered and hemorrhages are less apt to happen or are better controlled. Thus, no drainage tube from the bladder is necessary and the incision can be completely closed.

There is no question about it, this method does afford excellent functional results with lesser morbidity and allows earlier ambulation than with the supra-pubic approach... mainly because the bladder wall is not entered. It is generally recognized that by means of retro-pubic prostatectomy the patient feels less discomfort and the general improvement in the patient's condition is more rapid than in all other means of surgery to the prostate.

The hospital stay is usually shortened by this method and the prostate capsule heals quickly. There is little post-operative shock and the mortality rate in the hands of a good surgeon runs somewhere between 1% and 2%.

Perineal Prostatectomy

This means of prostatectomy has many advantages over the other approaches. Complete removal of all the hypertrophic tissue is readily permitted by this means. It permits much easier and more natural drainage away from the operative area and thus accumulations are not contained within a specific cavity.

This technique is especially suited where the large gland is situated lower in the pelvic cavity.

Hemorrhage is more readily controlled because of the direct vision involved.

Calculi and abscesses of the gland are more readily handled.

The danger involved in the perineal approach is danger to the rectal wall and to the external sphincter muscles. Thus it is

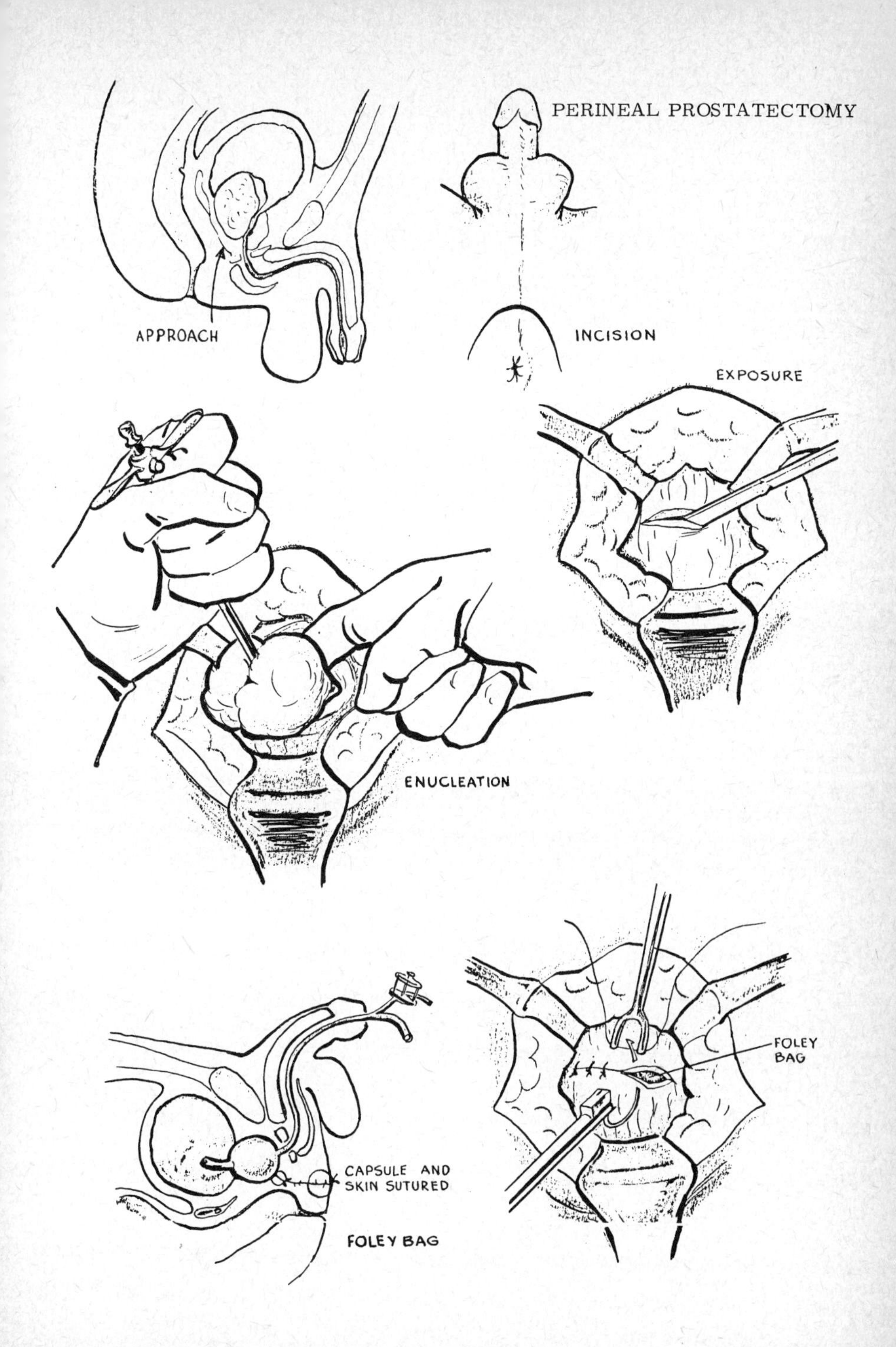

PERINEAL PROSTATECTOMY
APPROACH
INCISION
EXPOSURE
ENUCLEATION
FOLEY BAG
CAPSULE AND SKIN SUTURED
FOLEY BAG

considered a more difficult procedure than the other methods in this regard.

Further, it requires a more accurate knowledge of the perineal structures.

This operative method is definitely not suited where the individual is extremely obese or where the patient has limited hip motion. Perineal surgery should not be attempted on patients where the prostate is located extremely high in the pelvis.

When this method is correctly executed, there follows relatively little shock even in patients who are normally considered poor risks.

Entrance is gained by means of a semi-circular incision above the anus.

By this method, where the adenoma is unusually large, excessive bleeding may occur. But because of direct vision the hemorrhage can be controlled.

Healing is said to be the quickest by this method.

By far the most important advantage of the perineal approach is that suspected malignancies can be promptly biopsied ... and if it is found to be cancer, further surgery can be promptly effected.

Sex After Surgery

Here is an important fact that my studies have brought to light.

It is still possible for a man to perform and enjoy the sex act even after his prostate has been removed ... although the force of the ejaculation will be lessened or eliminated. However he cannot perform the sex act if his testicles have been removed or seriously damaged. You are probably familiar with the term "eunuch." This usually means a man who has had his testicles removed and is no longer capable of performing the sex act.

At this stage you might ask, "If a man can perform the sex act without a prostate, then why did nature provide him with a prostate? So why worry? At the first bout or sign of trouble have it removed!"

Well, it must be recognized that the prostate is a complex structure, being vital to both the sexual and urinary functions. In fact, it plays an important role in the control of the urinary flow, being related to the sphincter muscles of the bladder. Therefore, whatever affects the prostate will also affect the bladder, urethra, ejaculatory ducts, vas deferens ureters and ofttimes even the kidneys.

From the best information that I can gather it appears that the prostate supplies a secretion that carries the semen, when called upon, through the urethra and deposits it into the female by means of the ejaculatory process. Prostate surgery usually writes "finis" to the forceful ejaculation. Whether or not conception can ever take place once the prostate has been removed has not been proven. At least I have never read or heard of an instance where a man who has had his prostate removed sired an offspring ... and I have made wide inquiries.

Chapter Five

MODERN MEDICAL METHODS

To start with let me tell you of a most impressive bit of research in the field in which we are dealing. This interesting experiment was conducted by Drs. Julius Grant and Henry Fineblut and it was reported in the Journal of the Maine Medical Association, March 1958. This covers a controlled experiment in which 40 men with non-cancerous prostate enlargements were used.

Eighty per cent of the men were treated with glycine, alanine and glutamic acids. The prostate swelling decreased in 92% of the cases. In 32% of the cases the prostate returned to normal size. In 72% of the cases, discomfort was decreased.

Now concerning the other 20% ... these patients were given placebos or inactive capsules. They showed no comparable improvement.

For your information I would like to mention that glycine, analine and glutamic acids are found most abundantly in calf and chicken livers, lamb, beef and veal, as well as in kidney beans, brewer's yeast, peanuts and lentils.

The following is instructions to physicians, under Prostatism, from a handbook published by one of the largest drug houses in America:

Etiology and Incidence

Beyond the age of 60, enlargement of the prostate is found in 40% of men, half of whom have symptoms, which may be due to benign hypertrophy, carcinoma, or fibrosis of the prostate. The cause of benign hypertrophy or of carcinoma is unknown. Fibrosis may follow inflammation of the prostate but this is most common at an earlier age (30 to 50 years).

Pathology

Benign prostatic hypertrophy begins as multiple fibroadenomatous nodules which appear simultaneously under the epithelium of the posterior urethra. These enlarge concentrically, compressing the normal prostatic tissue laterally against the anatomic capsule of the prostate. This shell of normal prostatic tissue is the so-called surgical capsule. Rarely, the hypertrophic mass may push out into the bladder lumen as well, forming a pedunculated ball-valve type of 'middle lobe'.

Prostatic carcinoma arises in the posterior lobe adjacent to the rectum. It is unrelated to benign prostatic hypertrophy but sometimes occurs simultaneously with it. It most often is a slow-growing adenocarcinoma which penetrates the capsule of the gland and metastasizes to adjacent tissues and the bones.

Bladder infection, dilatation, trabeculation, diverticulum formation, calculus formation, hydronephrosis, uremia, hypertension and sepsis may result from prostatic obstruction.

Symptoms and Signs

Large congested prostatic lobes cause bladder irritability even before they begin to obstruct the urinary passage. Urgency, frequency and smarting may occur, although the stream still is normal in size. Partial urinary obstruction follows, with nocturia, increased frequency, incomplete emptying of the bladder, a small feeble stream and straining on urination. Bleeding may occur due to congestion of the prostatic lobes. An insidious onset over the course of several years may result in chronic retention with overflow dribbling and a developing uremia. Elevation of the blood pressure, cardiac decompensation and the mental confusion of early uremia must be watched for in the prostatic patient. Acute obstruction may ensue when the enlarged lobes become congested and completely block the narrowed outlet. This may be precipitated by ingestion of spicy foods or alcohol, attempting to hold the urine too long, exposure to cold, or immobilization in bed. Uremia (q.v.) is the consequence of continued back pressure and obstruction. Prostatic cancer produces urinary obstruction only after the entire bladder neck is invaded.

The stagnant residual urine behind an obstructing prostate easily becomes infected and increased frequency and dysuria then occur, together with chills, fever, nausea and vomiting.

Supra-pubic dullness or bulging of the distended bladder and enlargement of the prostate as detected by rectal examination (although intravesical middle lobe enlargements are missed this way) are the usual findings.

Diagnosis

Any male over 50 years of age with the above urinary symptoms should be suspected of prostatism. Patients in whom onset of the condition has been prolonged may fail to complain of obstruction, since they have forgotten what it is to urinate freely. Digital rectal examination usually will reveal an enlarged gland, but fibrosis of the bladder neck, median bars across the lower edge of the neck, or pedunculated intravesical middle lobes cannot be detected by rectal examination. Most prostatic cancers are readily detected by their enlargement, hardness and fixation. If the urine is sterile and has little or no pus in it, catheterization should be deferred until urinary antiseptics can be given prophylactically or until the patient canbe prepared for operation, should this prove necessary. A single catheterization then is permitted. Catheterization after the patient has tried to empty the bladder will reveal the amount of residual urine and also will reveal urethral obstructions. Catheterization also will indicate lengthening of the prostatic urethra in benign prostatic hypertrophy, since enlarged middle lobes make it necessary to insert the catheter almost to the hilt before it draws urine. Cystoscopy, best deferred until the patient is ready for operation, will demonstrate bars, fibrosis, enlarged intruding lobes, intravesical middle lobes, calculi, and bladder tumors. An I. V. pyelogram, NPN determination, ECG and chest X-ray are useful in evaluating the patient preoperatively. Urine concentration tests are the most accurate kidney function tests which are practical. Urethrograms taken in the oblique projection demonstrate the type of enlargement and may help to differentiate carcinoma from benign prostatic hypertrophy. The serum acid phosphatase rises only after a prostatic carcinoma has penetrated its capsule. X-ray of the pelvis and spine for osteoblastic metastases and biopsy of the prostate gland are other methods of differential diagnosis. All doubtful nodules which are confined to the prostate should be biopsied perineally or by needle, with the patient prepared for total prostatectomy should examination of the sections indicate carcinoma.

Complications

These include cystitis, vesical diverticula, calculi, prostatitis, pyelonephritis, hydronephrosis and hydroureter, renal insufficiency, and uremia.

Treatment

If symptoms are mild, if residual urine is under 3 ounces (90 cc.), if kidney function is good, and if there are no diverticula or calculi, palliative treatment is permissible. Congestion of the enlarged prostate may be relieved by the use of a hard seat or chairs and by avoiding cold, dampness, long rides in automobiles and trains, alcohol, pepper and other highly seasoned foods and condiments, and sexual excesses. The urge to urinate must be obeyed promptly and the bladder must never be permitted to become over-distended. Transitory difficulty in urination may be relieved by sitting down in a tub of warm water to urinate. Intensive therapy must be used to combat any infection which occurs. Inoperable carcinomas may be benefitted by castration or hormone treatment. Estrogens may cause slight shrinkage of the gland, but must be given for a period of 3 months or more. Testosterone propionate may increase the bladder tone slightly but it is definitely contraindicated in any case where the possibility of prostatic carcinoma exists. Prostatic massage with the evacuation of large amounts of prostatic fluid is of only the most transitory help.

Prescriptions

Diethylstilbestrol Tablets U.S.P. 1 mg.
10 tablets daily for 10 days; then
5 tablets daily for 10 days; then
3 tablets daily for life.

Ethinyl estradiol (tablets) 0.5 mg.
1 tablet daily for life.

I want my readers to take special note of the fact that the Diethylstilbestrol and the Ethinyl estradiol tablets are to be used for the rest of your life. From my knowledge of Diethylstilbestrol, as gained from many sources including the Merck Index, I know that Diethylstilbestrol will cause or can cause cancer as well as eunuchization of the patient. I am suggesting that Diethylstilbestrol will make it so you will have no sexual intercourse for the rest of your life. Of course, maybe it won't make any difference. But I am taking special pains to bring this to the attention of my readers.

In the author's sincere desire to give all possible forms of treatment of prostate conditions it was felt that the opinions of a noted Soviet urologist, Prof. E. M. Porudominsky, should be included among the Modern Medical Treatments. I am quoting ad verbatim from "Northern Neighbors":

We consulted Prof. E. M. Porudominsky, a noted Soviet urologist, and give his views on an ailment that afflicts many men, and affects wives also.

Here's what the Doctor says about

PROSTATE TROUBLE

For obvious reasons cancer of the prostate is not covered in this discussion, which is limited to "prostatitis".

*What is "the prostate"?

Dr. Porudominsky: The prostate, found only in men, is a gland that surrounds the neck of the bladder and the urethra (urinary canal), and consists not only of glandular but also of muscular tissue.

*What purpose does the prostate gland serve?

Dr. Porudominsky: Besides producing the spermatic fluid required in the act of reproduction, the secretions and nervous-system functions of the prostate play a very important part in male sexual life ... and thus, indirectly, in the life of women also.

*What is the ailment which men usually call "prostate trouble"?

Dr. Porudominsky: It is "prostatitis", which means "inflammation of the prostate". Contrary to popular belief, prostatitis is not a disease of old age alone, but is often found in younger men.

*Is there a definite known cause for prostatitis?

Dr. Porudominsky: Prostatitis may arise from many causes. Often an infection starts it. This may be gonorrhea, or non-sexual infection ... all kinds of common "strep" and "staph" infections, infections in the kidney and bladder, virus diseases such as influenza, etc.

*Then it really has nothing to do with sex life?

Dr. Porudominsky: On the contrary. Prostatitis can arise from non-venereal infection. But such infections can be passed on from women to men during intercourse. Also, prostatitis may arise from causes other than infections.

*Could you explain that statement, please?

Dr. Porudominsky: Abnormal sexual activity often causes inflammation of the prostate. For example, long-delayed or deliberately interrupted sexual intercourse, which prevents normal discharge of the fluids produced by the prostate, can lead to gradual enlargement and inflammation of that organ.

*What are the common symptoms of prostatitis?

Dr. Porudominsky: As a rule, prostatitis starts suddenly (from infection), is very painful, often with restriction of urine-discharge. But sometimes its onset is gradual. Dull pain, weakness, loss of appetite, insomnia, depression, headaches, these are common symptoms. I would like to point out that doctors -- even specialists -- often find the diagnosis of prostatitis a difficult one to make, because symptoms may correspond to a wide variety of other ailments.

*But doctor, is it not true that prostatitis is usually suffered by men in middle-age or later years?

Dr. Porudominsky: That is so. Infections, and abnormal sexual activity, are not the only cause of prostatitis. Soviet studies show that older men develop this disease not because of age itself, but because of a sedentary (sitting-down) life.

*Well! That is indeed interesting. Perhaps you can enlarge on that view, doctor?

Dr. Porudominsky: A life of physical idleness has a profoundly negative effect on the prostate. Mainly because of resulting poor blood circulation, but also because chronic constipation can start or worsen prostate gland disorders. Prostatitis we find most often in men who are in poor physical condition.

*But that is not the only common cause?

Dr. Porudominsky: The prostate is closely linked with the central nervous system, and that is why prostatitis can be caused by extremely exhausting physical or mental work, by severe strain on the nervous system, and, in some cases, by prolonged absence of sexual intercourse.

*Any other common causes, or associated conditions?

Dr. Porudominsky: We find that hemorrhoids (piles), especially if long untreated, can lead to prostatitis. So can diseases of the kidney and bladder. Many men neglect such ailments for years, and gradually develop prostatitis, which cannot be blamed on their age.

*Doctor, do you believe prostatitis can be prevented ... rather, can anything be done to avoid it?

Dr. Porudominsky: Most important is to completely clear up any and every infection, including "mild" infections such as flu. And of course any man with prostatitis should get immediate attention from a medical specialist, followed through by complete treatment.

*But aside from medical help, what other means?

Dr. Porudominsky: Above all, a strict routine that includes plenty of physical exercise, and adequate rest, is vital in preventing prostatitis. That's of greatest importance to men doing desk work. They must have sports, games, every day after work, and should exercise several times during the working day.

*How is prostatitis usually treated in the U.S.S.R.?

Dr. Porudominsky: First by curing such conditions as infection, hemorrhoids, etc. A wide variety of methods, of course, are used in such treatment. But many cases of prostatitis are treated by massaging the prostate gland. This should be done only under guidance of a specialist, because excessive massage is harmful. But it is often very beneficial -- improves blood circulation, tones up the muscles of the prostate.

*Do you use any other "physical" methods?

Dr. Porudominsky: We sometimes prescribe warm enemas. Another common form of treatment for prostatitis, in Soviet hospitals, is the warm "sitz bath" (water bath limited to hips). We insist upon total abstinence from alcohol and tobacco, which have a very harmful effect on prostatitis victims, and we prohibit riding bicycles or horses, until the disease is fully cured. Prostatitis can be completely cured by modern medical treatment.

Miracle Drugs for the Prostate

I'd just like to sound a rather strong warning against the false hopes raised by the so-called miracle drugs. I'm not trying to tell you that there are no drugs that can be of benefit nor do I decry the use of any drug or all drugs ... but I do wish to strongly advise that you seek other means and methods of help for your prostate condition without looking for or hoping to find a miracle drug.

Just a few years ago "testosterone" was heralded as the miracle drug not only for the prostate troubles but for many other conditions that cause trouble with male reproductive and urinary organs and glands. It received the most flagrant praise and ballyhoo of any drug put on the market. In fact, the manufacturers or the chemical company that made it evidently went to great ends to hire or procure the services of a well known writer who did a book on the subject and I had the unhappy displeasure to read the book. In any event "testosterone" did nothing but make a fortune and is still making a fortune for the manufacturer of that drug. But as for its benefits, I contend that it does more harm than good and is still doing a lot of harm.

So lest you be taken or led to believe that some miracle drug can help you or clear up or cure your condition, I am sounding this most emphatic warning.

Too, the reason I am stressing this warning is because not only will the drug or the so-called miracle drug delay your progress through other therapeutic means but you will also suffer various harmful side-effects, which usually follow in the wake of most drugs. I fully understand that if you are troubled with your prostate, you don't need the additional harm that the side-effects can create.

Furthermore, I am sure that some people may think that this warning is completely unnecessary. But having been troubled with a prostate disorder I feel that any warning that will prevent you from making an error and delaying needed action is well worth the effort.

Chapter Six

OLDER MEDICAL METHODS

While the treatment herein does not use drugs or medicine, I put it in this chapter because the author was a qualified M.D. Furthermore, his handling of the situation appears to be masterly and, therefore, I place it before you.

From the book "How to Treat the Sick Without Medicine," written by James C. Jackson, M.D., dated 1881:

"Urinary Disease -- The urine, as everybody knows, is a fluid secreted from blood. It is composed of excrementitious matter which, in order to the health of the body, it is necessary should be cast out of it. In all vertebrated animals, the bladder, therefore, is to be found, it being a cyst or bag into which the excrementitious matters held in suspension in the water of the blood are carried, and thereby cast out in the act of urination. From the very fact that the fluid is excrementitious, it is impossible in all cases to determine by it what the morbid conditions of the body at large may be. There is a class of physicians who style themselves Uroscopic doctors, who claim that they can, by the examination of the urine of any person, tell whether he is in health or sickness, and if sick, what is the disease under which he labors. In my earlier practice I gave a good deal of attention to the theory which these physicians set up, analyzing the urine of hundreds of persons, undertaking thereby to determine the nature of the diseases under which they suffered. But I found that the basis for diagnosis was altogether too narrow. And while it is true that one may, in many instances, come to very safe general conclusions in regard to the diseases under which certain persons suffer, the diagnostic basis is altogether too incomprehensive for general practice. The Uroscopians, therefore, have necessarily to confine themselves to special diseases, and hence cannot rise to eminence in general practice. For diseases of the liver, kidneys and bladder, the Uroscopic theory presents some advantageous considerations; but, on the whole, cannot be worthy of the regard which is claimed for it by its advocates.

"As far as my own practice has gone, I have found that urinary diseases, as a general thing, are secondary, the bladder and its adjunctive structures being unlikely to take on diseases belonging exclusively to itself and them. Idiopathic diseases therefore of the bladder and its auxiliary structures are seldom seen, unless arising from mechanical or physical injuries.

"More likely than otherwise, then, when there is disease of the bladder it is to be found as arising in, and dependent upon, disease of some other organs. One of the most common causes of urinary diseases is disease of the blood. When the blood is apparently healthy or ordinarily healthy, urinary disease will scarcely ever be found to exist, except from mechanical injuries of the bladder or its immediate auxiliaries.

"Inflammation of the bladder is generally a disease of its mucous lining. Disease of the neck of the bladder is either congestion, or inflammation, or suppuration of it. Where disease of the neck of the bladder exists, whether in congestion, or passive, or active inflammation of it, disease of the urethra or the canal through which the urine passes to expulsion is likely to exist. Many persons suffer from painful urination, the sensibility being at the outer termination of the urinary passage. This almost always indicates irritation or inflammation of the neck of the bladder.

"Aside from injuries, no person need have disease of the urinary organs, provided he lives within the line of temperateness in food and drink, and keeps the other organs of his body in such natural conditions as that they shall perform their functions properly. I do not think one person in five hundred thousand ever had disease of the urinary organs if he lived so as to keep the other organs of his body in anything like fair health. But where one eats like a glutton and drinks like a debauchee; where he dresses so as to check the external circulation, and relates himself to the action of the bowels so that these shall become necessarily unhealthy; where sedentary habits exist and imperfect clothing of the lower limbs is bad, and care and anxiety are constantly affecting his mental and moral nature, urinary disease may arise; and under such circumstances oftener than from any other set of causes do arise.

"What one wants, therefore, to do in the way of prevention, is to live hygienically, and whenever a case of disease of the urinary organs is clearly manifest, what one wants to do for its cure is to be treated psycho-hygienically.

"For inflammation of the bladder, when it is active or acute, one of the best things to be done is, having given the patient a thorough ablution, accompanied with good hand dry-rubbing, to put him upon a nitrogenous diet, keeping out of his food carbonaceous or heat-forming substances, to give him soft water to drink, and this only; to make him take a recumbent posture, and in the main to keep it; to lay upon his bowels over the bladder hot fomentation cloths, and keep them on until the pain, if it be acute, has sensibly subsided; then to keep upon him cool compresses all the time -- if he can bear them all around so much the better; to give him sitz-baths two or three times in twenty-four hours, while the acute manifestations exist, and the colder these are, up to the point where they do not feel uncomfortable, the better for him; to keep his feet warm by frequent rubbing of the hand, aiding the circulation, or else by wrapping them in heated flannels; to keep his head cool, and especially the back part of it, having preparations so made as to be able to lay wet, ice-cold cloths right in the nape of his neck once or twice a day; also to rub the whole length of his spine with ice-cold cloths, determining the circulation to the skin, and answering the ends of cupping; if this cannot be done by the application of cold cloths alone, then to have hot cloths laid up and down the back-bone, as hot as he can bear them, followed by cloths as cold as ice-water can make them, thus changing the circulation both of the blood-vessels and of the nervous system as much as may be. For where inflammation of the bladder comes on suddenly, being an acute disease it must be broken up as soon as it can be, even at the risk of some strain to the constitutional vigor of the patient. But where the disease exists in chronic form, having been long preceded by continued congestion of the bladder, either of its body or its neck only, and so has come at length to take on what might be termed passive inflammation, then there is less necessity for immediate executive results, in which case the better plan is to treat the patient generally as well as locally.

"Where chronic inflammation of the bladder exists, I have always found the wet-sheet pack to be one of the best remedial instrumentalities I ever used. In truth, if you can get up a very active cutaneous excretion, relief to the patient becomes almost immediately sensible, and though such relief does not argue positive cure, it does argue positive curability, and is a source of very great conscious comfort to the sufferer; for to carry about with one consciously such condition of the bladder as passive inflammation of it often establishes, is to be in about as uncomfortable a physical condition as one can be placed from any disease of any organ or organs of his body, where great and painful suffering is a constant attendant ...

"It also oftentimes may arise from piles, or from irritation in the lower bowel by small worms. Dysentery sometimes causes it, but, on the whole, more frequent causes are those which are to be referred to the state of the urine, arising, as a distinguished physician thinks 'From the nature of the ingesta, or from the changes consequent from primary or secondary assimilation of them.' Dr. Prout observes that 'Causes of irritability of bladder depend on functional derangement of the kidneys, usually resulting from the unnatural properties of the urine. Deviation from the normal condition of the urine, whether in deficiency or in excess, are recognized by the concomitant organs, and may prove a source of irritation in the bladder.' Dr. Copland says that 'The use of unripe fruits, especially by children, and often by adults, frequently occasions the complaint.' He also says that gonorrhoea and masturbation are among the most frequent causes of irritability of bladder.

"My own observation has led me to feel that however varied and influential may be the causes of producing irritability of the bladder, all others put together do not equal in influence and importance those which arise from the use of drug-medicaments. All the drastic purgatives which are prescribed by allopathic physicians tend directly to cause irritability of this organ. All the class of diuretics particularly are so calculated, and whenever I find a patient of mine to have fixed irritability of the bladder, I am quite as much disposed to search for the cause, direct or remote, in the use of some drug-poison which he has been taking, or is taking, as in any other direction.

"My practice, therefore, with this disease, even when it is seen in the form of incontinence of urine in children, or indicated by the want of power to retain urine in any considerable quantity by adults, is so to change the action of the general system as to remove, as far as may be, the more obvious causes of irritation. Hence, a change in regimen is of great import. I should never think of allowing a patient of mine who had irritability of bladder, and who wanted to urinate every half hour, or as often as every two hours, to eat flesh meats at all; nor should I permit him under any circumstances, except such as should be adjudged purely transitional, to use common salt. The use of this substance, I think, is very provocative of the disease; and wherever the disease exists, while it is used it utterly precludes cure.

"I recollect not long since of meeting a gentleman who was troubled with irritability of bladder, not being able to contain more than a gill, and generally not more than half a gill of urine without being painfully desirous to micturate; a man of pretty full habit of body, living highly, and therefore having a good deal of waste matter in twenty-four hours to pass out of his system through this great excretory. He had either to undergo great pain, or else to pass water as often as once an hour, or not infrequently, under great mental excitement, as often as once in thirty minutes. He had consulted various physicians, and they had foolishly given him diuretics, supposing, in their mistaken notions of his case, that what ailed him was a want of secretion of urine. He got no relief from them. Under the use of some of their medicines he was made worse. Meeting him, he begged the privilege of stating his case to me, saying that although he didn't know much about my methods of treatment, he had heard of me frequently, and would like to state his case to me. I said to him I would be very glad to give him any information or advice that I could. So he told me how he was affected.

"Curious enough, although he was quite a user of spirituous liquors, a great tobacco chewer; was not, by any means, sexually continent, and approximated nearly to the state of the glutton in the indulgence of his appetite for food, my suspicions, under his description of his case, were awakened, particularly with respect to his use of common salt, and so I said to him:

"'Do you use common salt?'

"'Well, yes,' said he, 'I eat quite moderately of salt.'

"'How much do you eat?'

"'Well,' said he, 'you know these little salt-cellars that are on the tables of hotels; I suppose I eat two or three of those full at a meal.'

"Now, that any man should do so and yet think that he did not eat much salt, surprised me. I said to him, 'I think you will find yourself greatly relieved by a substantial disuse of salt; in fact, if you could do without it entirely, I think in one month you would be very greatly benefitted.'

"He said he could. And he did.

"I saw him about three months after, and he came to me and took hold of my hand, and the tears stood in his eyes while he said, 'You cured me. I do not suffer at all. I sleep all night. I have not eaten a teaspoonful of salt in ninety days.'

"The poor fellow had been suffering for years in this way, and the more he suffered, curious enough it was the more salt he had come to eat. In this case, the simple disuse of the irritating substance cured him.

"I am very glad to be able to say that distinguished physicians of the allopathic school agree with me in their views of the hurtfulness of animal food, especially where persons have what is termed the gouty rheumatic and uric-acid diatheses; and that they also consider that malt liquors and spirits are still more injurious, and that wine is of no service whatever."

A Pathologist's View

Here I cite from a letter I received from an old experienced pathologist in answer to my inquiry concerning his views on prostate conditions:

"Enlarged prostate is made out as if it occurred in every male after a certain (unspecified) age. I did not see many cases in the autopsy room (1910-1914). I make out it has nothing to do with sexual activity, for quite a number of cases I have heard of (coming for operation to St. Mary's Hospital) were elderly priests.

"I have had inquiries on 'how to prevent', because there are ads about this very commonly. Knowing where to get such information I have sent for pamphlets, but I do not think they are any good; the layman knows no more about it than the doctor, though he may think so. The surgeons make out that large prostates are early or actual 'cancer', hence must be removed. I personally had a prostatectomy six years ago; was told it was the largest they had ever seen (!), but I kept it at bay for years by a homoeopathic remedy (Saw Palmetto); and could have gone on longer but for getting a 'flu' attack one February: had to go to hospital to get relief as evidently no one uses a catheter nowadays; so of course when they found out the size thereof, it had to be removed -- since when I have had no more anxiety about micturition (of course).

"I think that is about all I really know about the subject. Those who have had large families get enlarged prostate about the same as those who have had small ones, or those who are bachelors."

A General Practitioner's Attitude

This is a communication received from an old highly respected medical doctor in Quebec who replied to my inquiry as to how he would treat a case of retention of the urine due to prostate disorder:

"If a man comes to me in the middle of the night with acute retention of urine, and it is almost always in the middle of the night, the first problem is to give him relief.

"First you try a soft catheter size 18F. With a gloved finger in the rectum to guide it over the prostate, you are usually successful. If not successful, which sometimes happens, you give him a hypo. of morphine 1/4 to relax his tension, because tension and straining to urinate forces the prostate down into the urethra thus acting like a ball valve.

"Sometimes the morphine alone is sufficient to make him relax and urinate; if not, then you use a stiff coude catheter #18. If this is not successful you try a metal sound, which is a steel instrument with a curve that you can guide over the prostate with your gloved finger.

"With this instrument you need great care and gentleness, otherwise you may make a false passage up behind the bladder as happened to me. Then you are in real trouble.

"If you are near enough to the hospital you put the patient in your car and take him there. If you are too far away you use a trocar and drive it into the bladder just above the pubis. This I also experienced.

"In the hospital, after three days on antibiotics to control possible infection and under anaesthetic, the surgeon inserts a cystoscope into the bladder to look around and look for cancer. He may find that it is simply a prostatic bar across the outlet of the bladder, in which case he will scoop out a passage through it into the bladder and insert a Foley catheter to control bleeding as well as to not let the passage he had made heal up worse than before.

"He will also take a punch biopsy of the prostate, especially of any lump that he may feel. This together with what he has removed by surgery he will send to the pathology lab to be examined for cancer. This is done while you are on the table, and the surgeon waits. If it proves to be cancer the surgeon will do a supra-pubic prostatectomy and later treat you with deep X-ray or cobalt. If he finds no cancer he may stop there but if the prostate is very large, he may do a prostatectomy anyway, depending on his own convictions.

"In this case the whole gland will be sectioned and examined for cancer.

"As for treating a large prostate without surgery I know of no treatment; although I have often wondered why they cannot shrink the gland with deep X-ray or cobalt bomb. Even Dr. Koch, Dr. Krebs and Dr. Beard do not claim success with Glyoxylide or Laetrile.

"I put a great deal of faith in the Anthrone

Test for cancer as done by D . Howard H Beard of Forth Worth, Texas."

I quote this next section for three reasons: (1) the volume is fifty years old, having been published in 1915, (2) because of the eminent authorities who authored it -- Oliver T. Osborne, M.D. and Morris Fishbein, M.D. and Jerome H. Salisbury, M.D., (3) because the information, although more than 50 years old, is in some ways as pertinent today as it was then ...

"If there is no residual urine, good; sensible tonic treatment, a proper amount of rest, a properly regulated diet, good management of the bowels, prevent of chilling, and the happy medium of never attempting to hold the urine too long or on the other hand answering every frequent flitting desire to urinate, may hold the patient in the same condition for months or even years. It is undesirable to allow the patient to urinate too frequently, because it prevents the bladder from becoming normally distended, and the viscus becomes smaller and smaller until life becomes a misery."

"If there is residual urine and this (which may vary in amount from day to day) persists from day to day, it is only a question of time when the patient will have a sudden stoppage and be unable to empty the bladder and must send for a surgeon for immediate catheterization on account of distention of the bladder with resulting paralysis. This having once occurred, some surgeons advise the use of a catheter continuously. It is possible in such an instance that if a proper attendant with the most careful cleanliness uses the catheter at least three times in twenty-four hours, and perhaps better four times, in a few days the bladder may return to its proper tone and may be as good or better than it has been before for a number of months, i.e., may not contain so much residual urine. This should be tried. If, on the other hand, the bladder does retain residual urine, and the urine tends to be alkaline and turbid, the man must be given a catheter to use himself, either once in twenty-four hours to remove all residual urine, or three times in twenty-four hours if he cannot at any time well evacuate his bladder. This kind of treatment is sometimes necessary on account of the inadvisability of operating, but is generally inexcusable, as it is only a question of time when such a bladder will become seriously infected and chronic cystitis, incurable, will be the result, and cause the death of the patient. Therefore, unless there is some positive reason why a man cannot be operated on, operation should be advised before infection has occurred.

"Some patients develop a chill after the passage of even a soft rubber catheter, or even have what has been called the urethral fever, with considerable rise of temperature for some hours. This is not of frequent occurrence, and may never be seen by an individual practitioner. Other surgeons have seen it so frequently that they recommend the administration of some drug to prevent this hyperirritability of the urethra, such as bromids, and even quinin has been recommended. If such a reaction occurs, the patient should be kept in bed for twenty-four or thirty-six hours and treated symptomatically. No harm seems to come from the disturbance."

Chapter Seven

TREATING PROSTATIC HYPERTROPHY W TH VITAMIN F

Vitamin F in the Treatment of Prostatic Hypertrophy

By
James Pirie hart, B.Sc.
and
William LeGrande Cooper, M.D.
Los Angeles, California

Received for Publication August 1, 1941

For a considerable time we have been using an oral vitamin F complex preparation for the control of the common cold. This treatment has been used quite successfully in Europe for several years. During the courses of treatment with this preparation it was noted that in certain male patients who were being treated concurrently for prostatic hypertrophy, there was a sudden notable decrease in the palpable size and consistency of the prostate gland.

This led us to investigate separately the

action of vitamin F complex on a series of cases of prostatic hypertrophy. However, before proceeding with our material, a necessarily brief survey of the nature of vitamin F might be in order.

Kugelmass summarizes the information as to the nature and composition of the product:

> "This fat soluble growth factor consists of the unsaturated aliphatic acids essential for normal nutrition. It is a common constituent of animal fat, and is 'associated with' the linoleic or linolenic fraction. Vitamin F is essential for cell respiration, insulin secretion, epidermal synthesis and hair metabolism, other lipid functions being fulfilled by dietary fat."
>
> "... A residual amount of vitamin F persists in the liver even on a diet free from unsaturated fatty acids, although absent in body fat, the most potent sources are egg, lard, linseed oil and corn oil."

Evans and Lepkovsky found that:

> "Vitamin F, unlike vitamins A, D, and E, is not concentrated in the non-saponifiable fraction. It can be recognized in the fatty acid portion after saponification."

Sherman finds that the purer forms of unsaturated fatty acids do not exhibit the same F effects as natural oils high in unsaturated fatty acids.

Numerous observers have proved that there are definite, deleterious effects upon experimental animals and the human organism, when these unsaturates are deleted from the diet. Upon return to a diet containing these factors the organisms demonstrate marked restoration to normal.

The majority of workers are of the opinion that these unsaturated fatty acids, in certain combinations, undergo synthesis in the body, perhaps in the liver, converting them into the typical vitamin form. Shephard believes the reaction may take place in the skin.

Clinical Procedure

The total number of cases in our report is nineteen. Six other cases were deleted due to failure to continue treatment or to cooperate. Laboratory blood determinations were made of five patients taken at random from the group.

Our procedure was as follows:

1. The gland was palpated to determine its size and consistency.
2. A residual urine was obtained.
3. A detailed history was taken of the urinary symptoms regarding force of stream, spraying effect of stream, dribbling, nocturia and cystitis.
4. Each patient was given a thorough physical examination for the exclusion of other vitamin, mineral or endocrine deficiencies.
5. Blood samples were obtained for the determination of lipids, iodine, calcium, and phosphorus.

We did not check androgen levels but we believe further investigations will yield interesting information in this respect.

Patients were then placed on a daily dosage of six five-grain tablets of vitamin F complex, a concentrate containing linoleic, linolenic, and arachidonic acids, each tablet having a total of 10 milligrams of these unsaturated fatty acids. This dosage was administered for a period of three days to produce systemic saturation; it was then reduced to four tablets daily for several weeks; finally a maintenance dose of one or two tablets was administered daily.

Physical examinations were given each month, at which time blood samples were taken for determination of essential change. The patients also reported weekly for observation of their subjective symptoms.

Results

1. All cases showed a diminution of residual urine; in 12 of the 19 cases there was no residual urine at the end of the treatment.
2. Nocturia was eliminated in 13 of the 19 cases showing this symptom.
3. A decrease of fatigue and leg pains and increase in sexual libido was noted in all patients.
4. Cystitis cleared up in relation to the decrease in residual urine.
5. Dribbling was eliminated in 18 of the 19 cases.
6. Force of stream was increased.
7. In all cases the size of the prostate was rapidly reduced. Confirmation was by palpation.

Every patient exhibited enthusiasm over the improvement in physical well-being resulting from treatment. The few showing the least improvement had all given histories of gonorrheal infection of varying degrees of involvement of the genito-urinary tract.

Laboratory Findings

In essentially all of these cases our laboratory findings indicated low blood lipids, high or normal blood calcium, and low blood iodine at the start of the treatment. Tissue lipids, tissue iodine and tissue calcium were low, as was to be expected. Shortly after treatment was instigated a notable reversal of the above factors was observed in the laboratory specimens.

Five patients were taken at random from nineteen cases. The period of treatment varied from ten days in Case No. 5 to forty-five days in Case No. 1. (Compare figures of "before" and "after" Vitamin F Therapy as given on Page 320)

Although this is a small number of cases the results are so consistent that the following conclusions may be drawn:

1. Blood calcium showed an average decrease of 11.2%.
2. Blood phosphorus showed an average increase of 8.3% under the same conditions.
3. Blood iodine increased 307.3%.
4. The striking increase in the blood iodine content after vitamin F therapy suggests a strong functional relationship between this vitamin and the thyroid gland.

Before Vitamin F Therapy

Case No.	Date	Ca (1)	P (1)	I (2)
1. J.P.H.	9-16-40	9.00mg	3.8 mg	5.5mg
2. R.L.	11-26-40	8.70mg	1.25mg	5.5mg
3. W.F.C.	11-22-40	9.50mg	2.60mg	10.0mg
4. H.H.B.	12-14-40	9.40mg	2.20mg	8.5mg
5. K.W.W.	12-23-40	10.30mg	1.89mg	4.0mg
Averages		9.38mg	2.35mg	6.7mg

After Vitamin F Therapy

Case No.	Date	Ca (1)	P (1)	I (2)
1. J.P.H.	1-4-41	7.10mg	3.93mg	16.5mg
2. R.L.	12-26-40	8.40mg	1.79mg	22.5mg
3. W.F.C.	1-6-41	7.70mg	2.98mg	32.0mg
4. H.H.B.	1-4-41	9.00mg	3.50mg	26.3mg
5. K.W.W.	1-4-41	9.00mg	1.94mg	11.7mg
Averages		8.24mg	2.83mg	21.8mg
Differences	Increase		0.48mg	15.1mg
	Decrease	1.14mg		
Percentages	Increase		8.3%	307.3%
	Decrease	11.2%		

* Ca (1) and P (1) - Milligrams of calcium and phosphorus per 100 cc. blood serum

* I (2) - Micrograms of iodine per 100 cc. whole blood

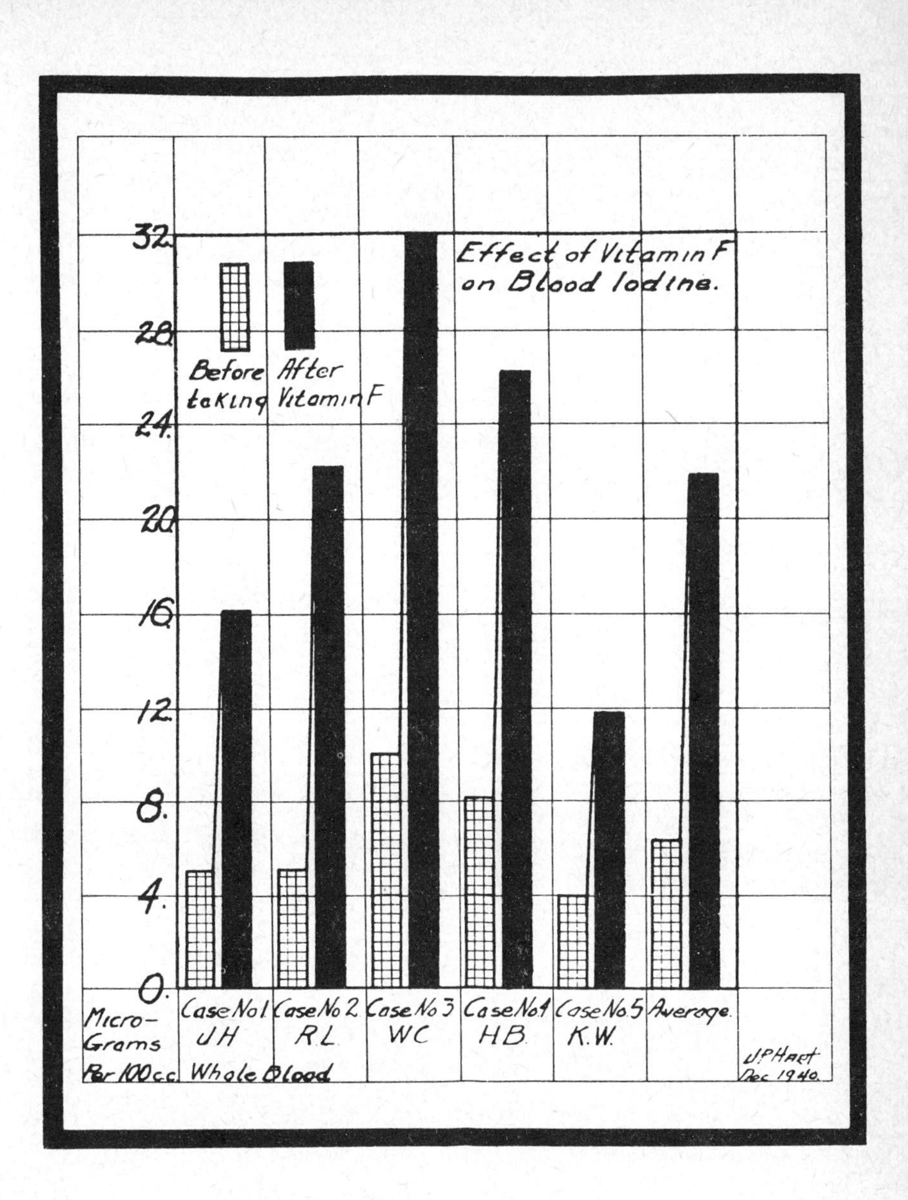

EFFECT OF VITAMIN F ON BLOOD IODINE

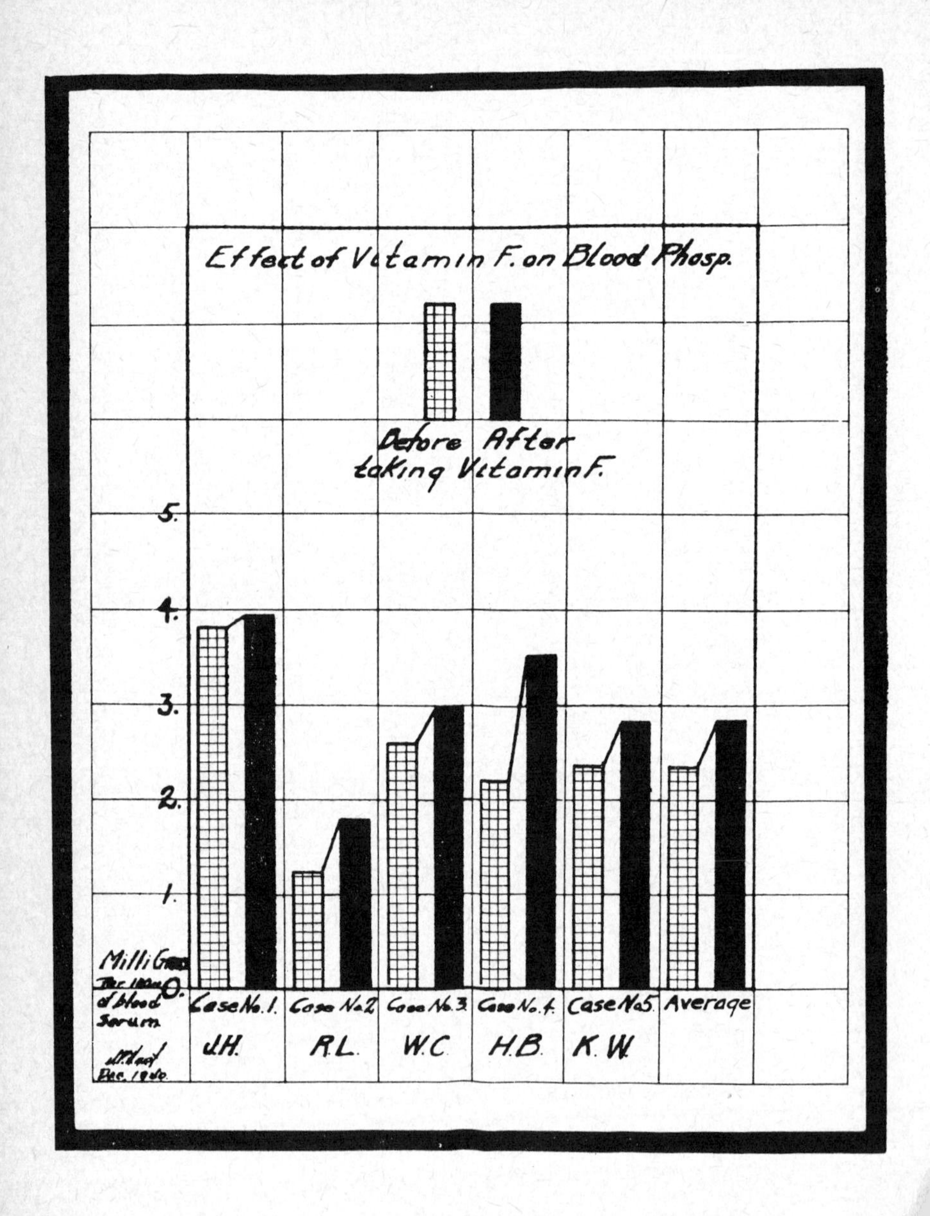

EFFECT OF VITAMIN F ON BLOOD PHOSPHORUS

hostile environment and man's evil habits, and the symptoms of these ailments should not be treated and suppressed."

While the treatise on the hygienic system appears to be the shortest and the simplest, its virtues should not be taken lightly or ignored. Because of its simplicity one may doubt or pass it by. I beg you not to make that tragic error.

There are a few capable hygienic system practitioners in America. Their treatment not only consists of fasting but most important, the system demands the teaching of proper eating and living habits. These practitioners will prevail upon you to practise and learn their system of eating and living. While undergoing treatment and following the fast, I stress, they use neither drugs, medicines, potions, herbs or manipulations.

Chapter Ten

WHEAT GRASS METHOD OF TREATMENT

This treatment has been suggested, prepared and written by Anne Wigmore, D.D., the originator of the "Wheat Grass Method" and the "Wheat Grass Manna Drink." Many people in all walks of life can attest to the efficacy of her treatment for various conditions.

"We seek to rebuild the entire body while we are making definite efforts to reach the organ involved in the most direct way.

"First: We insist that the sufferer adopt our simple diet in order to bar 'unsuitable' food from the body -- the food that caused the prostate trouble in the first place by sending too much acid into the urine. Also, with this 'unsuitable' food barred, Mother Nature can work with the great variety of LIVE nutrients -- the minerals, vitamins and trace elements found in the FRESH juice of the wheat grass chlorophyll -- UNDISTURBED and UNHAMPERED.

"Second: We insist that the sufferer take at least three three-ounce drinks of freshly-squeezed out wheat grass juice each day, spaced conveniently away from meals. This enables Mother Nature to reconstruct the blood stream and send healing substances into the affected prostate.

"Third: We insist that the sufferer, at least three times a day, shall 'implant' in his rectum at least a half glass of freshly-squeezed-out wheat grass juice -- propping his abdomen up, on pillows or a slant board -- so that the liquid can come as close as possible to the prostate gland and be partially absorbed through the tissues. This is our direct attack. And it works.

"We have never had an unfortunate with prostate trouble whether chronic or acute that did not respond favorably to this three-ply method. In many, many instances, operations that had been scheduled, were abandoned by the medical doctors who had heretofore believed that they were vitally necessary.

"In addition, we try to have the sufferer, on arrival at 'The Mansion', go on a three day wheat grass fast prior to the intensive methods described above, to clear the intestines of waste matter -- eating between the wheat grass mannas, a few grapes minus the skins, if hungry. This seems to prepare the digestive organs for the simple diet which is to come and hastens the effective healing work."

Chapter Eleven

YOGI THERAPY FOR AN ENLARGED PROSTATE

Here it is as described by a well known practitioner from India and prepared especially for inclusion in this volume:

"As all disorders in the body culminate from incorrect eating and living habits, the yogi will prescribe a regime of purifying methods such as fasting for three days or more so as to give the organism the opportunity to cause an elimination throughout the system including the obstructed organ such as the prostate. After the fast, the patient will be advised to live largely on the fresh non-stimulating fruits and vegetables in place of cooked foods, and animal foods such as meat, fish, eggs and cheese. In other words to forego the eating of salt and other substances which may produce acids and toxins in the system which will help to retain fluid in the system. The fruits and vegetables that the yogi will prescribe will be those that are non-irritating or pungent and which mostly ripen above the ground in the rays of the sun. In other words, the more spicy or condimented foods such as garlic, onions, mustard, horseradish are best omitted.

"From the yogic point of view, complete healing is only possible through strengthening all weakened areas of the body. As the body is a complete unit a series of exercises will be given which will improve the nerve and blood supply to the entire system -- such exercises are like the shoulder stand, the plough, the cobra, and many of the other exercises which twist the spine in various positions, stretch the limbs, loosen the joints, and improve in every other way the postural poise of the body. In addition to these exercises for the harmonious development of the body specific exercises for the affected or flaccid organ are such exercises which will directly tone up and normalise by a period of contraction or tension which is followed by a period of relaxation. Possibly the simplest and most effective in this group is the mula bandha which merely amounts to the contraction of the anus and lower sections of the rectum. If this is practised correctly one will definitely stimulate and improve the blood supply to the prostate as well as to the urethral passage and muscles surrounding it. An exercise which can supplement this is uddiyana bandha, and nauli.

"Mula bandha is the static version of aswini mudra, which is the contraction of the sphincter-muscles of the anus. This latter bandha is necessary to prevent the air which is locked within to escape through the rectum, while uddiyana bandha (the drawing

in of the abdominal cavity towards the spine) creates an internal pressure which assists in the retention of the breath.

"Uddiyana bandha. One must be capable of drawing the abdomen in and out fifty times on one exhalation. With a short rest between rounds, thirty such rounds must be completed at one session so as to reach 1,500 contractions. By toning up the vital organs contained in this viscera which is really the motor of the body, digestion is improved, constipation is overcome, and the psychic import of the body is heightened through the nerve centre contained in this region.

"Nauli is the basic exercise for basti, dauti, vajroli mudra (sex control), and the awakening of the serpent power kundalini. It is best executed in the morning on an empty stomach in a standing position, although it can be performed while sitting in padmasana. Stand with legs apart, hands on thighs, and body leaning slightly forward. Commence by exhaling all the air out of the lungs to practically the last vestige -- after which draw the abdomen inwards and upwards. The hollow cavity now attained is called uddiyana bandha which is the first stage towards liberation according to yoga terminology.

"Aswini mudra is best practised after nauli and uddiyana bandha have been perfected. When undertaking this mudra take a position on the knees and elbows, and after exhaling, by the use of the will contract and relax the rectal muscles. While doing this visualize that you are drawing the anus and navel together. This mudra controls the apana gas (which is free of odour), and has an additional function of having a beneficial influence on the concentration of nerve endings situated in that area. Once this is perfected a tube is not required to allow water to pass into the rectum when doing basti.

"Additional measures are the use of the hot and cold sitz baths. The hot bath used at night to dilate the urethra and so permit the retained urine to be voided. The cold sitz bath used in the morning will contract the urethral passage so that this area will be given added tone.

"Please note that the yogi system gives special attention to the endocrine system because centuries ago they realized that the glands are the important transformers in the body which manufacture from the blood flowing through it the important hormones, glandular extracts and essences needed for vital living. The sexual glands, such as the prostate, are given extra attention because they reproduce the secretions for procreation as well as for internal rejuvenation.

"This briefly gives the yogi method in a nutshell."

Chapter Twelve

NATUROPATHIC METHODS

Here I am quoting a letter from a friend of mine who is a highly respected naturopathic physician:

"If retention is complete and acute, I would first have catheterization performed so as to make the patient as comfortable as possible.

"It is of great importance to remember that each case presents its own individual problems and the care that is given is adapted to each case individually.

"My procedure usually is to discontinue all solid food for about three days, placing the patient on fluids, plain water, fruit juices, hot vegetable broth or any of the herb teas, about 8 ounces every 2 to 3 hours or when hungry. I also suggest lukewarm water enemas daily and a hot epsom salt bath every evening before retiring as well as plenty of sleep and rest and relaxation. In some cases the baths and enemas for the first few days may be used twice daily, morning and night.

"I further insist that these patients keep

their feet warm and follow a regulated program of exercises adjusted to their particular needs and make-up.

"After the first three days the diet adjusted to the individual case may be somewhat as follows: one kind of fruit for breakfast; small vegetable salad with cottage cheese or ricotta cheese or one steamed vegetable, or any fresh fruit with cheese for lunch and raw vegetable salad, baked potato and one steamed vegetable for dinner. Later, small portion of lean fish or chicken or any lean meat is permitted in place of baked potato, about 2 to 3 times a week.

"All spices, condiments, sweets, cookies, pastries, ice-cream, artificial beverages, coffee, tea, and liquor, are eliminated, and smoking is discontinued.

"This procedure has proven highly successful in many cases but will not eliminate the need for surgery in some cases, especially where the prostate has grown so large and hard that it can no longer be reduced, and the obstruction is not lessened.

"Also, even where no complete obstruction exists we must make sure that there is no excessive urine retention since this may ultimately back up and cause kidney damage.

"In these cases I usually insist that no fluids or fruits loaded with fluid be taken after 4 p.m. and that the patient be careful not to eat too much food when taking the last meal of the day.

"If I am called to a case where

catheterization is not urgent, I try the enemas and baths first to see whether I can induce urination. If catheterization is urgent to empty the bladder, then this should be done first and the program followed to see whether urination normally, cannot be brought about.

"Occasionally, even with the best of care, the prostate may have become so large and hard that shrinking it and relieving the obstruction is impossible. Then you have no alternative but to turn the case over to a qualified surgeon. However, the program outlined usually provides relief ... and this gives us an opportunity to carry on by natural means to rebuild the patient's health.

"What is important to stress is that even when urine retention is relieved, the prostate is still large and hard and carelessness in our mode of living may bring about a return of the original difficulty. In other words, a very careful program of living and care must be followed continuously.

"Another point to remember is that in these cases, the prostate involvement is usually only a link in the chain of various other involvements -- endocrine imbalance, general tension, nervousness, often arteriosclerotic changes, arthritis symptoms may be found and even if the original urinary retention is brought under control for the time being, unless the general health is rebuilt, recurrences of the problem can be expected."

One of the veterinarian surgeons whom

I consulted re prostate conditions in animals passed on to me this interesting bit of information which I am passing on to my readers:

"Prostate or any other disease is caused by malnutrition in animals or man. The proper treatment is to remove the cause. In most cases patients return to good health unless the disease has destroyed one or more of its organs.

"A raw potato suppository is soothing to the area and very likely furnishes some nourishment by absorption. I don't know of any disease that would not benefit by garlic therapy. It is a food for man or animals. Garlic oil capsules per rectum is a specific for local irritation, whether it be for babies, dogs or cats.

"Fenugreek is like garlic, goldenseal and marshmallow. It is good nutrition and is almost always beneficial. I have used marshmallow myself and recommended it to men who report 'it's wonderful'."

The treatment for prostatitis by a naturopathic physician in South Africa:

The best approach to the condition is first by drainage of excess acids from the body (particularly the pelvic area) through fasting, pelvic massage, spinal manipulation, alternating hot and cold sitz-baths and dieting. The subsequent diet should be vegetarian-fruitarian for at least two or three weeks before introducing mild proteins that are easy on the digestion. Brains, tripe, veal, a little white fish (steamed or baked) are suitable for this purpose. A purine-free diet is always beneficial.

Sunflower seed oil -- about one dessert-spoonful daily either neat or with the salad meal -- is very beneficial. Foods containing zinc are thought to be beneficial to prostate cases.

As almost all cases will be elderly the fasting should not be longer than one day to a week according to the actual age. Patients over 75 years of age should not fast more than two days at a stretch.

Until the condition is well on the mend distilled water is the only kind permissible. Cold sitz-baths are very effective and essential in most cases.

Rectal massage is merely a temporary relief measure.

Before retiring each night the prostate patients should take a fairly hot sitz-bath for a period of five minutes and release the bladder contents into the bath if urination was impossible before sitting in the tub. Take no liquids after 5 p.m., daily. Take a cold sitz-bath on arising each morning. The hot-sitz will dilate the urethra and the cold-sitz will contract it. When urination is still difficult or impossible these sitz-baths should be alternated, i.e., one minute in the cold and then three minutes in the hot. Repeat this three or four times until a full and free urination is achieved.

Chapter Thirteen

CHIROPRACTIC TREATMENT

Prostatitis

Submitted by a lecturer at one of the Chiropractic Colleges

This title is a broad term which is used indiscriminately by most persons to include a few infectious processes, still more cases which are an endocrine imbalance and a great majority which are primarily cystitis. Because of this we must make a few clarifications.

Any frank infectious process has a resulting inflammation which will leave the prostate swollen, moderately soft and quite tender. The swelling usually causes obstruction to the urine flow and the inflammation spreads into the bladder to cause further irritability so the person usually feels like they have to void very frequently, for a very small amount. The obstruction, however, causes a marked delay in starting the micturition.

The endocrine imbalance is quite

common to most men past forty years old, with a gradual hardening occurring in varying degrees so that in the extreme stages there is a marked delay in both starting and stopping urination. This is not accompanied by inflammatory reaction so there is no irritability and the constant desire to void. The majority who are diagnosed as prostatitis usually have a simple uncomplicated cystitis, in which any bacteria found are usually incidental contaminants. There are some frank bladder infections, but most cases of cystitis are not frank infections. With this inflammation of the bladder the prostate can be entirely unaffected so there is a great desire to void quite frequently, but there is minimal delay in the initiation of micturition or voiding the urine. Since there is little obstruction to bladder evacuation, this is one of the primary symptomatic differences, which is frequently overlooked.

Chiropractic care of patients who have been diagnosed as prostatitis will depend entirely upon the proper diagnosis of the cause of the condition. It is a well established fact that bacterial infection can only follow lowered tissue resistance. Therefore, the value of the chiropractor is most important in the preventive phase of health maintenance. If the person has become extremely run-down and has a severe frank infection, the chiropractor upon recognizing this condition, will refer the patient to a urologist who specializes in these conditions and may be able to administer the appropriate chemotherapy. In order to appreciate the approaches to the endocrine imbalance and to the simple cystitis, it will be necessary to briefly discuss the background of such conditions.

There was a time when the endocrinologists considered their specialty to be fairly well isolated from that of neurology since they looked upon each of the endocrines glands as supplying an optimum secretion to maintain the proper balance between all these glands. That viewpoint was similar to describing an excellent orchestra but without any conductor. At the present time however, the endocrinologists have adopted a new title so their official publication is now entitled Neuro-Endocrinology. The immediate inference is that the orchestra does need a conductor and the co-ordination is obviously made through the nervous system. This is even more obvious when we consider a statement of Prof. Zondek, who is often considered the Dean of the Endocrinologists when he stated "the hormones circulate in an unactivated form and perform their specific function only at the point of destination." Recent experiments with deep general anesthesia have shown however, that even insulin has no effect on blood sugar while the nervous system is under deep general anesthesia and thereby unable to make its response to the hormone. It is well known that adrenalin has a great effect on the clotting time of blood in a living person with normal nerve response, but the same adrenalin has no effect on the clotting time of the same blood in a test tube. Therefore, it becomes obvious that the nervous system must be functioning normally in order for the endocrine glands to do their proper work. It is apparently through this mechanism that many patients have had good results in rebalancing the endocrine system while under chiropractic care without the use of any hormone therapy whatsoever. In this light, then the reversal of the aging process on the prostate gland following proper chiropractic care is very closely related to the response of the diabetic patient who has found that his blood sugar level has changed so much that his medical doctor had to discontinue the use of insulin after the patient had chiropractic correction for a spinal problem which was upsetting the nerve supply to the pancreas. Like other pathologies these endocrine imbalances do have a less favorable prognosis for each year of duration. Glandular tissues can degenerate and become eventually replaced with scar tissue from which there is no recovery under any form of treatment.

The "prostatitis" which is usually a simple cystitis is primarily a neurological problem in which the lining of the bladder becomes unduly irritated with the passage of the usual irritants within the urine. Since the urine is a waste product of the body it contains varying amounts of many different poisons, crystals and other materials which would be highly irritable to skin or mucus membrane in any other area of the body. The lining of this urinary tract has many sensory nerve endings which keep the central nervous system aware of the state of affairs at that location. Similarly minor cuts, scratches and bruises elsewhere on the skin heal up very well with minimum attention, when the person is healthy. So also are the minute repairs done consistently in the lining of the urinary tract in response to the various sensations arising from these terminal endings. This is very much like keeping up one's house with the patching of little cracks in the plaster, replacing the washers in the faucets and replacing the light bulbs as they are exhausted. If a person did nothing about keeping up his own house (for two year's time) it would soon become a junk heap. The same thing happens various places in the body when the sensory nerve supply has altered from its normal response. When the repairs are not kept up, the lining of the bladder becomes highly irritable and may enter a rapid break-down stage. A similar mechanism will allow a joint to disintegrate and crumble apart quite painlessly if the sensory nerve supply has cut off. Part of the same mechanism is responsible for the slow healing of wounds and the ulcer formation in a person with diabetes. When the sensory nerves are not responding as they should in minute injuries the repair processes are neglected and the whole structure disintegrates rapidly. In a very minor and diffuse form the same mechanism is the basis for most cases of simple cystitis which are often mis-diagnosed as prostatitis. The question then arises as to how the sensory nerve supply can be disrupted. Fortunately, these warning signs do arise before there is a total disruption and the symptoms usually appear only at the time when the information coming from these sensory endings is only slightly "out of tune" as it is received by the central nervous system. At this stage chiropractic care is usually very effective.

Fortunately, the Doctor of Chiropractic has been taught to consider pathology as not the final scar or tumor or ulcer which is the end result; but rather the abnormal action in the physiology which is leading toward this end result. It is quite logical to assume that one does not go from normal tissue to scar tissue immediately, but most go through the intervening stages of inflammation, degeneration and finally replacement with scar tissue. Therefore, the chiropractor is not compelled to wait until the last stages of the disease become incontestable before he can begin applying correction to the abnormal process. It is well known for example, that in the early stages of any disease with fever whether measles, polio or flu, there are certain common symptoms, but there is no way in this early stage of distinguishing pathology which would develop in a few more days. At this early stage even the best specialists could not distinguish the three conditions which two days later became very obvious even to the average layman. In this way chiropractors have handled many, many conditions in which a final diagnosis was never made because the malfunction became normalized before the classic symptoms developed. Therefore, you will find that a chiropractor does not treat prostatitis or cystitis, but rather attempts to correct the cause which is usually an imbalance of the function of the nervous system.

Abnormal functioning within the nervous system which is usually the major problem with cystitis and which you so often find mislabelled prostatitis, can be any one of three different problems. First there can be a dietary indiscretion which is either depriving the body of its proper nutrition or is adding a great deal of excess irritant to the urinary tract. Second there may well be continued stress, physical or emotional. Emotional problems with a sense of insecurity in many individuals arise in present society. The third factor in the nervous irregularity is that of direct trauma to the body which can and does, frequently cause a subluxation in the spinal column with direct damage to the nervous system. These three conditions occur in varying combinations and it can be complicated further by bacterial contamination. Therefore, the responsibility is just as heavy on the medical doctor to rule out the possibility of spinal subluxations before giving medication as it is for the chiropractor to rule out the possibility of frank infection before he attributes the problem primarily to that of spinal correction which is his specialty. Fortunately the present day chiropractor is adequately trained to make this differentiation and to realize very clearly which cases fall in the realm of chiropractic and which cases fall within other fields.

The chiropractor is thereby faced with the problem of first making a comprehensive case history, to enquire into the dietary habits as well as the patterns of emotional distress with a particular individual. The chiropractor will then make a comprehensive spinal examination and locate any possible causes of disturbance with the nerve supply to the bladder and the prostate. He may then begin correction of the obvious faults in the spinal column or if they appear to be minimal he may well have more intensive examination done on the prostate and the urine to rule out frank infection. Since a patient does not become sick in one spot while perfectly alright in every other place, it is only logical to consider the individual as an entire person and not just another case of prostatitis. For this reason the chiropractor will not only make the necessary spinal corrections, but will also point out to the patient the many different things which he can do for himself in the way of avoiding undue stress, both physical and emotional, of the necessity of good dietary habits and of the many other little simple things the patient can do to help himself. If there has been a severe direct injury of the low back it may well be that the patient also needs some corrective exercises in order to strengthen the weak area just as corrective exercises to strengthen a sprained ankle are essential in the proper recovery. For a person with habitual bad posture there may well be the necessity of additional self-administered exercises in the way of correcting the weight-bearing problem which may well have been a big factor in the original spinal failure. There are many individuals who have been standing with a sag in the low back so many years that they have a constant backache, primarily due to the poor posture of which they may be totally unaware. Other persons may have developed a very similar poor posture due to injury in that low back many years before and must now have not only advice on postural change, but also have chiropractic correction of the faulty spinal mechanics. It may now be much more obvious as to why the chiropractor will admit that some patients coming to him with prostatitis, cystitis, or both, have had excellent results but at the same time he will claim that he definitely does not treat either of the conditions as such. For this reason it becomes quite obvious that chiropractic education does include the necessary differentiation of the many conditions, not with the intent of making a final autopsy diagnosis, but rather concerned with whether the patient can be benefitted best with chiropractic care or whether he should be referred to another specialist. The chiropractor does recognize that there are many factors entering into the development of a pathology, but that throughout all these stages of any pathology the nervous system is drawn intimately into the process. The chiropractor is well aware that he does not have the "panacea" and is obviously not going to help every patient, but any condition which is predominently of nervous character responds exceptionally well to chiropractic care. The general public may not be aware of the relationship and many persons have never thought of prostatitis or arthritis or influenza as having any response whatsoever to chiropractic. Perhaps this discussion will help in the understanding of this problem.

"Prostatitis" under chiropractic care therefore becomes much more clearly delineated. A chiropractor will obviously send a frank infection to the urologist for the appropriate chemotherapy. The remaining endocrine imbalances, the nervous incoordinations and the simple cystitis which is very frequently called prostatitis will therefore be evaluated in the light of chiropractic care. Other factors in the general stress pattern are recognized but particular attention is directed to the spinal mechanics, as they directly affect the function of the nervous system. A chiropractor, like any other health practitioner will also try to have the patient help himself as much as possible in avoiding further aggravation of the problem, doing his best to cooperate in the correction. On the basis then, that both the motor and the sensory nerve supply to the various structures of the body can be appreciably altered by faulty spinal mechanics, the chiropractor is doing a competent job in contributing to the general public health. For this reason you will find many individuals across the entire continent state without qualification that their prostatitis was cleared completely when they were having chiropractic care. Rather than argue and try to completely clarify the issue many chiropractors will finally admit that they have "treated prostatitis," but if they have more time for a complete explanation they will almost always insist that they definitely do not treat any pathology, but are rendering chiropractic care in order to normalize body mechanics with its effect on the nervous system. Due to the complexity of the nervous system and due to the varied combination of past injuries of each patient, chiropractors find that there is no stereotyped approach which will work best with every individual. The most critical area in the spinal column may be approached directly with mechanical adjustments at that location, or handled at best at other times through reflexes in the nervous system as sensory stimuli some distance from the immediate symptomatic area. In this way chiropractors, specializing in apparently contradictory methods of approach, may get equally good results with patients having similar problems. The central theme of any chiropractic correction however, is in the normalization of the integrity of the nervous system through its interrelationship with the spinal mechanics.

In summary all "Prostatis" is not necessarily frank infection. The majority of cases are other types and after being differentiated with their cause properly evaluated the chiropractor has had many excellent successes with this type condition through his own peculiar specialty of working with the nervous system, by the route of normalizing the spinal mechanics. In this way a person can see where chiropractic care has a much broader scope than just that of backache.

Chapter Fourteen

AYURVEDIC TREATMENT (FROM INDIA)

In severe retention of the urine, due to enlargement or other disorders of the prostate, apply any good vegetable oil on the lower abdomen (the pubic area) below the umbellicus ... followed by hot fomentations on the same area or a hot tub bath.

According to Ayurved, enlargement of the prostate is due to long standing bad food habits -- especially foods lacking in proper oils and fats -- and irregular habits of elimination.

Chapter Fifteen

THE AUTHOR'S COUNSEL

Everywhere, but everywhere -- in newspapers, magazines, periodicals, promotional literature and over the radio and television stations -- we are given advice about health ... but there is usually a footnote or an introduction that says, "Caution: Wherever any difficulty arises concerning your health, it is advised that you at once consult a physician and place yourself completely under his care."

I am suggesting that if this is your inclination why by all means consult your medical doctor or the healer of your choice. However, my experience and my intellect tell me that in many cases there are other means that would be as good or even better.

I do not believe that such an added warning is either necessary or justifiable. To suggest that whenever you have the slightest headache or trouble you consult your doctor is nothing but drumming up business or free advertising for the healing professions and drug and chemical enterprises.

Nevertheless, I want to express clearly and emphatically that there are some wonderful doctors and healers in many fields and some mighty capable surgeons who do remarkably fine work. But that does not necessarily mean that one has to run to a medical doctor whenever he has an itch in his bum or a tickling in his testicles.

Remember, today we no longer have the vacant-corner-lot medicine man of the last century, with his entertainment and ballyhoo and big spiels. There are no longer untrained, unqualified, unlicensed healers to filch the public. The M.D.'s, chiropractors, osteopaths, naturopaths, medical herbalists, the Christian Scientists and the Faith Healers are all licensed and controlled. Furthermore, the literature disseminated by any healer is quickly brought to the attention of the powers that be. I don't think there are any dangerous unlicensed practitioners of the healing arts running around loose and free ... at least not in the part of the world in which I reside.

Let's face the simple truth ... there are many people who are opposed to the taking of harmful, caustic, searing, synthetic chemical drugs and refuse to have them put into their bodies whether by means of a shot, a toxin, a vaccine or any other way. They have the inherent right and they should have that right ... to choose the practitioner of their choice, be he drug, drugless, manipulative, layer of hands, voodoo or otherwise. They should furthermore be allowed to treat themselves if that is what they want to do and what they believe in.

A man has but one life to live or lose and if he wants to abuse it, I don't think there is anything that you or I or anyone else can do or should do about it. There is no more justice or logic in compelling a man to consult a medical doctor if he has the bellyache and wants to take a dose of castor oil, than there is in compelling a man to hire a contractor when he wishes to build a house or in compelling a man to seek the services of a gardener if he wishes to dig a few trenches in his garden.

There is no doubt in my mind that doctors do receive an excellent training and education along their prescribed and accepted lines, but it must be remembered that this intense training is on all matters pertaining to disease. Their training is never in health or how to gain or maintain it. Keep this vital fact in mind.

It is my belief that very few healers in any or all of the healing professions can distinguish between an over-distended bladder and a prostatic condition. I have tried with all my power to check this matter out with many practitioners in many fields and I am left with the conviction that few if any healers can positively distinguish the one from the other ... unless the patient undergoes a cystoscopic examination, which only a urological surgeon can perform.

Invariably, when you go to a healer with an over-distended bladder or retention of the urine, your condition is immediately diagnosed as prostate trouble. Of course, the digital examination -- that is, through the rectum -- will quickly reveal the oversized prostate if it exists ... and as I said before, about 75% of all males over 50 have an enlarged prostate anyway. If it is found that the prostate is enlarged, immediately all else is ignored and the prostate gland is blamed for all the trouble. I urge you to give consideration to the fact that the whole urino-genital tract is involved and the cause of the enlarged prostate may be one of many things. Remember, in the urino-genital tract there are many organs, among them being the kidneys, ureters, bladder, prostate and the urethra. I contend that close and more careful consideration should be given by all the healing professions to the entire urino-genital tract as well as all-round body health before assuming that the prostate is infected or is causing all the trouble.

It is admitted that the prostate may be enlarged or even grossly enlarged but that does not mean that it is the cause of the trouble. It may be and I sincerely believe that the prostate is but the victim ... the goat ... and that its enlargement is due to overwork beyond its normal capacity. Therefore, removing this important gland will not necessarily remove the cause of your trouble.

Patience, study and the avoidance of causative factors at a time like this may indicate that the prostate is not entirely or at all to blame ... but is just the victim. Further, it must be borne in mind that an over-distended bladder can cause enlargement or other disturbance of the prostate ... and trouble with your kidneys.

Make no mistake about it ... there frequently comes a time when the urologist performs a most vital role. Thousands of men alive today would have been dead had it not been for the skill of the well-trained urologist. Just ask anyone who came to the end of his tether, because of procrastination or on account of many forms of self and other treatments, and who at last found relief at the hand of a urologist ... what he thinks of his urologist!

It is not my intent to sing the praises of and tell you how wonderful are the urologists. I want to counsel you with all my powers of persuasion to change your living and eating habits so that you can live and urinate without having to come, as a last resort, to a urologist in desperation to save your life.

My suggestion is that anyone who wishes to follow the natural treatment for prostate disorders should place himself in the hands of a capable naturopath -- a practitioner who believes and follows the teaching or way of life known as 'natural hygiene'. However, if the sufferer is unable to do this, then the following instructions are given for his benefit.

To begin with, it is absolutely essential that the sufferer completely re-organize his way of living and his daily habits. It must be understood that the changing of habits is of prime importance and also that this is a most serious and time-consuming procedure. Usually prostate troubles do not show up until one has reached the 4th, 5th or often the 6th decade of life and by then most habits have become deeply ingrained and to change them at this stage is difficult, to say the least. Yet, if you wish to overcome prostate difficulties by natural means without drugs or surgery or manipulation of any kind, the change must be effected. I beg you to understand that I am deliberately making it sound difficult so that you will not allow yourself to think it is a cinch.

For the first few days -- at least 3 days -- I would suggest avoiding all solid foods and restricting the intake to only water. Drink ample water but do not drink so as to distend your bladder. Three or four days or even longer on a water diet should do nothing but good for any normal human being. I would not advise fasting beyond this period unless you place yourself under the supervision of a qualified practitioner.

Copious water intake should be continued during the day but after 4 o'clock in the afternoon it should be stopped to avoid distending the bladder while sleeping. Upon arising in the morning, the intake may be resumed.

Some may suggest the use of fresh juices at this time. I would urge you to restrict yourself to fresh, natural water. No sweetening or any other agent should be added.

After the third or fourth day one should go off the fast by taking 4 ounces of fresh carrot juice every two hours and as much water as desired, but at least 3 or 4 glasses a day. Follow this juice diet for one day ... but once again, no fluids after 4 p.m. Then for the next two days stay on a raw vegetable diet.

Fresh fruit diets exclusively are recommended by many naturopathic healers for the natural treatment of prostatic trouble. I would definitely recommend the use of a strictly vegetable diet -- no fruits of any kind for the time-being -- and of course, all uncooked.

The use of all alcoholic beverages must be given up immediately. Coffee, tea and soft drinks must also be eliminated from the diet. However, if this is impossible or too difficult, then at least all beverages should be restricted to an absolute minimum ... but absolutely no coffee! Some people in their drinking habits will use as many as 10 to 20 cups of tea, coffee or other beverages in a day. If you must drink, drink water ... cold, warm or hot. By using any beverage except water you are definitely placing an undue strain upon the kidneys and to a lesser extent also upon the bladder, the prostate and the urethra. It would be wise to restrict your liquid intake to fresh vegetable juices and ordinary untreated water.

I doubt very much if total success will crown your attempts to alleviate prostate troubles unless you give up the use of all harmful beverages. The only other beverage that I would permit in addition to water and fresh fruit and vegetable juice would be natural herb teas, restricted to 2 or 3 cups a day without sugar, milk or cream.

The diet should consist preferably of raw vegetables and after a few days, fruits. Go extremely light on all heavy protein foods. Drink at least four 8-oz. glasses of water a day. For the first few days I would suggest omitting all forms of flesh foods from your diet.

Salt, that is table salt in any form, should be definitely eliminated.

For the sake of exercise and body tone the friction bath is recommended -- that is, a dry friction bath with a rough towel over the entire body. Also, take part in as much physical exercise as you can stand. Do as much walking as possible, as many miles a day as is practical.

Because the prostate gland is located adjacent to the rectum, an enlarged prostate and a full rectum can cause irritation which may lead to undue pressure and a feeling of fullness in the rectal area. Continued congestion in that area and in the tissues surrounding it can be a source of serious trouble and discomfort. Under no circumstances should force or pressure be brought to bear upon the rectum, by forcing or straining at stool in order to procure a bowel movement. Because of the danger that may arise under this set of circumstances, many healers believe that enemas are essential. This means of emptying the bowels should only be resorted to if there is no other way. But if there is no discomfort I cannot see the rhyme or reason for using an enema. Some people are too prone to making use of this unnatural form of bowel emptying.

If an enema is used -- and there are often times when there is no other way -- it should be used with care and deliberation. It should be small -- not more than a quart of water and preferably a pint -- and the water should be warm and injected slowly and gently into the lower bowel and retained only long enough to permit the proper evacuation. It is my positive belief that under no circumstances should any salt, soap, oil or other matter be put into the enema water.

If there is a choice between taking a laxative or purgative and taking an enema, the enema would be preferable for it would be less harmful. While most people can take an enema themselves, it is better and wiser if someone proficient in the art performs this task for you.

There are other healers who recommend colon irrigation, often referred to as 'colonics', for prostate and other ailments. This is strictly a matter of choice. However I do not feel that colonic irrigation is desirable, necessary or warranted. The recommended fast should, without fear of harm and complications, take care of the problem of evacuation.

Many of the old-time medical doctors, as well as other healers, have used this internal water treatment as a means of reducing the congestion in and around the prostate gland. The method followed to lessen the pressure is to inject into the lower bowel some 16 to 20 ozs. of water every day before retiring. Cold water is recommended. The water is injected very slowly just as you would an ordinary enema. The water should be retained in the rectum as long as possible, even for periods exceeding 30 minutes. Beneficial results can be apparent within a week to 10 days. However, the treatment can be continued on alternate days for a month or more. Please remember that nothing, not even salt or soap, is to be put into the water.

Many authorities feel that the above outlined water treatment is the simplest of all therapies and the least likely to be harmful. They claim it has helped and comforted countless thousands.

It is my belief that localized treatments are of little or doubtful value, except in cases of total retention. The over-all picture of the health of the individual must be the factor that decides the method of treatment.

Prostatic massage through the rectum is definitely not advised in the nature cure treatment. There are other schools of healing, including many physicians, who practise and recommend the palpation and massage, which I definitely do not advise.

There appears to be a great deal of controversy concerning the value of massaging the prostate gland. This is a practice that has been in vogue for many, many years and generally it is one of the first things that a physician used to do as a means of giving relief to his patient. Many still follow this practice.

J. H. Tilden, M.D., a famous old-timer physician and writer, has this to say about the practice of palpation of the prostate:

"Much injury is done this organ by massaging it, a treatment that is quite a fad among a certain class of medical men. This treatment is often as far-fetched as giving digitalis or strychnine for an already jaded heart, or morphine for a restlessness brought on from oxygen starvation in pneumonia, or for precordial oppression when the heart is aerated, or for headache due to the hyperemia of the brain. There is a difference in the results, however. The drugs used in such haphazard fashion often cause death, while the massage cultivates an enlargement of the prostate; or perhaps I should say that the massage becomes an ally of venery, coffee, tea, alcoholics, tobacco, sugar, meat and starch in hastening a senile tendency.

"Manipulation of the prostate is one of the hundreds of nonsensical professional innanities. The average human being is inexcusably gullible toward the titled, decorated profession; and the profession, being made up of the same common clay, do not hesitate to park their wants on a common so succulent."

Ad mentioned above, this practice is widely followed by many physicians but my studies reveal that there is no rhyme or reason for massaging the prostate. I know of one physician who had quite a following and earned quite an income just by this one type of treatment. Once this practice begins it becomes habit-forming for the patient finds it a vital need to have his prostate massaged regularly. I know that investigations will reveal the truth of these statements.

Another authority says: "I do not employ and do not approve of prostatic massage. Indeed any irritation of the prostate, whether in massaging it or examining it; or by treating it with injections and electricity, may and often does make the condition worse. Rough handling in examination and in massaging the prostate has been responsible for much mischief."

From a "Manual of Urology" by R. M. LeComte, M.D., F.A.C.S., written under the heading of "Local Treatment" and a sub-heading "Prostate and Seminal Vesicles":

"Massage is the method treatment most commonly applied directly to the prostate gland and is useful in subacute and chronic inflammations. It is accomplished by gentle stroking of the gland with the index finger, protected by a rubber glove or finger cot with shield; and inserted into the rectum of the patient. Whether the stroking motion is from the lateral borders to the center or from the upper to the lower margin is immaterial provided the pressure used is light and the manipulation not prolonged. Rough or too vigorous massage may bruise the gland and induce an acute reaction which may eventuate in acute prostatitis or seminal vesiculitis or in epididymitis. It is ordinarily repeated no oftener than twice a week. The purpose is to improve the circulation and to milk out secretion which might otherwise be retained. After the prostate has been massaged, the seminal vesicles may be emptied by stroking very gently once or twice along their course from without inward. The manipulation is completed by gently emptying the prostatic urethra by stroking from above downward."

Merck says: "Even the gentlest massage of the infected prostate or seminal vesicle may cause an acute and dangerous exacerbation with dissemination of the infection."

Prostatic massage is related by more and more authorities to be without any benefits whatsoever but it is recognized that it can cause harm. Just how much harm it can cause is not established.

One authority claims that it has been positively known for well over fifty years that massaging the prostate only aggravates the prostate trouble.

Pertinent advice to those who have had prostate surgery, as well as to those about to have it:

1. Avoid sexual intercourse for at least three months after surgery.
2. Avoid all alcohol beverages for at least 60 days after surgery.
3. Include a large vegetable salad with at least one of your meals a daily.
4. Go easy or better still, lay off coffee. It is definitely harmful.
5. Do not drink anything before retiring. Let your evening meal beverage be the last till morning.
6. Be sure to urinate within fifteen

minutes after indulging in sexual relations. Never go to sleep following sexual relations without urinating. Otherwise you may have a difficult or painful time urinating in the morning.

There is some controversy as to whether or not a man whose prostate has been removed can father an offspring. I maintain that a man whose prostate has been enucleated can cause conception to occur. As long as the gonads and seminal vesicles have not been removed or harmed, conception can take place.

By enucleating the prostate only the motility of the semen has been affected. The prostate, by means of the forceful ejaculation, hurled the semen out of the urethra and into the vagina, upwards towards the uterus. Thus, with taking time and care and by a practice akin to milking after the climax, the sperm can be aided in finding its way into the vaginal orifice. In this manner conception may take place.

It is recognized that most men past fifty have sired their families and are more pleased than sorry that they can no longer make a woman pregnant ... as long as they can enjoy coitus. However, a younger man who has had his prostate removed might possibly still like to be able to procreate.

Most men come through prostate surgery without incident. The mortality is very low -- somewhere around 1%.

Now that the problem of urination and its attendant complications have been eliminated why not keep it that way? To return to your old or normal pattern of eating, drinking and living will without the faintest doubt bring, if not a recurrence of your old problem, at least something as bad or worse.

Even while in the hospital undergoing the surgery and subsequent treatment I changed my eating habits and have maintained that change or even improved upon it. For example, I gave up coffee, tea and all beverages except a simple herb tea and hot water with a jigger of milk.

I scrupulously avoid any food that has an additive of any kind in it, be it coloring agent, flavoring agent or preservative.

Upon checking with innumerable people who have had prostatic surgery, I find that I have fared as well as the best and much better than most. Practically all seem to have some problem -- slight or major -- but all of them have one thing in common... they have returned entirely to their pre-operative habits and way of life.

I appeal to you, if you must have a prostatectomy or if you have had a prostatectomy, change your eating, drinking and living habits to conform to a natural or hygienic way of life and you will forestall many health problems or threats to your health. Forewarned is forearmed!

GLOSSARY OF TERMS

Acini -- Cluster, as grapes.

Calculi -- Stone-like masses which may form in the body under abnormal conditions.

Carcinogenic -- Causing cancer.

Carcinoma -- Particular type of cancer.

Catheter -- Tube for passage through body channels, usually to evacuate fluids.

Celibate -- One who is unmarried or practises celibacy.

Chemical caponization -- Castration by means of chemicals.

Coagulates -- Clots, as blood.

Coitus -- Sexual intercourse.

Coitus interruptus -- Removal of organ before ejaculation.

Coitus praecox -- Premature ejaculation.

Coitus prolongatus -- Prolonging the act by various means.

Coitus reservatus -- Without discharge of semen.

Condom -- Rubber covering worn over the penis to prevent conception.

Cowper's glands -- Two small bodies beneath the anterior part of the mucus membrane of the urethra, and opening in the bulbous portion.

Cystitis -- Inflammation of the bladder.

Detrusor -- An instrument used to displace.

Ejaculation -- Ejection of semen.

Eneuresis -- Incontinence of urine.

Engorgement -- Excessive fullness.

Enucleation -- Removal of a tumor or an organ in its entirety.

Estrogen -- Female sex hormone.

Etiology -- Study of the causes of disease.

Fistulae -- Abnormal passages leading from the surface of the body to an internal cavity.

Foecal -- Pertaining to foeces.

Gland -- A bodily organ by which secretion is carried on.

Gonorrhea -- Venereal disease.

Hypertrophy -- Increase in the size of an organ or part due to increased nutritive activity.

Incontinence -- Lack of restraint.

Indwelling catheter -- A catheter left in position for a period of time.

Meatus -- A passage; the opening to a canal.

Micturition -- Act of passing urine from the bladder.

Neoplasm -- An abnormal growth.

Nocturnal emission -- Involuntary ejaculation during sleep.

Onanism -- Complete sexual intercourse with ejaculation outside the vagina. Masturbation.

Orgasm -- Sexual climax.

Orifice -- Opening, entrance.

Palpation -- Examination by feeling.

Pathology -- Science that treats of diseases, their causes, symptoms, progress and results.

Perineal -- Between the anus and the scrotum.

Polyuria -- Excessive secretion and discharge of urine.

Posterior vesicle -- The hinder vesicle.

Prostatectomy -- Excision, complete or partial, of the prostate.

Prostatic urethra -- Part of urethra that passes through prostate.

Prostatism -- All disturbances connected with urination and obstruction of the bladder neck.

Prostatitis -- Inflammation of the prostate gland.

Proximal urethra -- Part closest to the point where the urethra originates.

Renal insufficiency -- Insufficient kidney function (kidney derangement).

Retro-pubic -- Back or behind the pubic area. Lower part of abdomen.

Seminal vesicles -- Vessels that store the semen.

Sitz bath -- Therapeutic bath in sitting position.

Spermatozoa -- Germ cells of the male.

Sphincter -- Muscle that surrounds and closes an opening.

Stricture -- Narrowing of any tube in the body.

Subcervical -- Below the neck of.

Supra-pubic -- Above the groin.

Transurethral -- Passing through the urethra.

Uremia -- Poisoning from urinary substances in the blood.

Ureters -- Tubes leading from the kidney to the bladder.

Urethra -- Tube which carries urine from the bladder to the outside.

Urologist -- Medical specialist who deals

with organs producing and transporting urine.

Uterus -- Womb.

Verumontanum -- The crest of the urethra.

BIBLIOGRAPHY

Volumes

ALVAREZ, Walter C., M.D. -- Review of Modern Medicine

AMIEL, M., N.D. -- The Prostate

ANDERSON, W.A.D., M.A., M.D., F.A.C.P. -- Synopsis of Pathology

BENEDICT LUST PUBLICATIONS -- Prostate, natural method of healing

BERG, Ragnar -- Vitamins

BICKNELL, Franklin, D.M., M.R.C.P. and PRESCOTT, Frederick -- M.Sc., Ph.D., A.R.I.C., M.R.C.S. -- The Vitamins in Medicine

BLOCH, Ivan, M.D. -- The Sexual Life of Our Time

BOWERS, Edwin F. -- Know Your Prostate

BRUBAKER, Albert P., A.M., M.D., LL.D. -- Text Book of Physiology

BURNET, R.W., M.D. -- Foods and Dietaries; A Manual of Clinical Dietetics

BODANSKY, Oscar, M.D., Ph.D. -- Biochemistry of Disease

CABOT, Hugh, M.D., F.A.C.S. -- Modern Urology

CHANEY, Margaret S., Ph.D. and AHLBORN, Margaret, M.S. -- Nutrition

CHETWOOD, Charles H., M.D., LL.D., F.A.C.S. -- The Practice of Urology

THE CIBA COLLECTION OF MEDICAL ILLUSTRATIONS, Vol. 2 -- Reproductive System

THE COLUMBIA ENCYCLOPAEDIA

THE ENCYCLOPAEDIA BRITANNICA

CLEMENTS, Harry, N.D., D.O. -- Prostate Troubles
COOPER, Lenna F., B.S., M.A., M.H.E., Sc.D. -- Nutrition in Health and Disease
DAVIS, Oliver Bennett -- Sex, Love, Longevity and Health
DE KRUIF, Paul -- The Male Hormone
ECKEY, E. W. -- Vegetable Fats and Oils
ELI LILLY & Co. -- De Re Medicina
EVERETT, Millard Spencer -- The Hygiene of Marriage
EXCELSIOR MEDICAL CLINIC -- Non-Surgical Treatment of Prostate Rupture and Hemorrhoids (Piles)
FISHBEIN, Morris, M.D. -- Modern Home Medical Adviser
FOSTER, M., M.D., LL.D., F.R.S. -- A Text Book of Physiology
FRIEDENWALD, Julius, M.D. -- Diet in Health and Disease
GOLDFIELD, Edwin D. -- Statistical Abstract of the United States (1966)
GREER, Joseph H., M.D. -- Sex Science
GROVES, Ernest R. and GROVES, Gladys Hoagland -- Sex in Marriage
HAVIL, Anthony, B.A. -- The Technique of Sex
HEALTHFUL LIVING DIGEST -- Gaining Health from Herbs and Foods
HELINE, Corinne -- Healing and Regeneration Through Color
HICKMAN, Cleveland Pendleton, Ph.D. -- Physiological Hygiene
HIRSCH, Edwin W., M.D. -- Prostate Gland Disorder

JACKSON, James C., M.D. -- How to Treat the Sick Without Medicine
KAUFMANN, Dale W. -- Sodium Chloride
KENYON, Herbert R., M.D. -- The Prostate Gland
KLEIN, Leo, D.C., Ph.D. -- You Are Not Alone
KLEINER, Israel S., Ph.D. -- Human Biochemistry
KLOSS, Jethro -- Back to Eden
LAKE, Thomas T., N.D., D.C. -- Treatment of the Prostate by Physical and Manipulative Therapy
LAMBERT, Gilles -- Conquest of Age
LEPP, Ignace -- The Psychology of Loving
LEWIN, S.A., M.D. and GILMORE, John, Ph.D. -- Sex After Forty
LIBER, B., M.D., Ph.D. -- Your Mental Health
LUCAS, Richard -- Nature's Medicines
LUST, Benedict, N.D., D.O., D.C., M.D. -- Universal Naturopathic Encyclopedia Directory
MACANDREW, Rennie -- Life Long Love
MACANDREW, Rennie -- Rennie Macandrew's Encyclopedia of Sex and Love Technique
McCANN, Alfred W. -- The Science of Eating
McCORMICK, J.H., M.D. -- Century Book of Health
MACFADDEN, Bernarr -- Man's Sex Life
McCOLLUM, E.V., Ph.D., Sc.D. and SIMMONDS, Nina, Sc.D. -- The Newer Knowledge of Nutrition

McLESTER, James S., M.D. -- Nutrition and Diet in Health and Disease
MEDICAL RESEARCH COUNCIL -- Vitamins: A Survey of Present Knowledge
THE MERCK INDEX -- Seventh Edition
THE MERCK MANUAL -- Ninth Edition
Miscellaneous Author -- Prostate Gland
OLIVER, J.H., N.A.M.H. -- Proven Remedies
OSBORNE, Oliver T., M.D. -- Handbook of Therapy
PHILIPP, Elliot E., M.A., M.B., B.Chir., F.R.C.S., M.R.C.O.G. -- From Sterility To Fertility
PIERCE, Dr. R.V. -- The People's Common Sense Medical Adviser
POMERANZ, Dr. Herman and
KOLL, Dr. Irvin S. -- The Family Physician
POWELL, Col. A.E. -- Food and Long Life
PRINCIPLES OF INTERNAL MEDICINE -- Second Edition
RAMACHARAKA, Yogi -- The Science of Psychic Healing
RANDOLPH, Paschal Beverly, M.D. -- Eulis Affectional Alchemy
RODALE, J.I. -- The Complete Book of Food and Nutrition
ROGERS, E.E., M.D., C.M. -- The Philosophy and Science of Health
SANGER, William W., M.D. -- The History of Prostitution
SANSUM, W.D., M.D. -- The Normal Diet and Healthful Living
SCOTT, Geo. Ryley -- The Quest for Youth
SHERMAN, Henry C., Ph.D., Sc.D. -- Chemistry of Food and Nutrition

SINDONI, Dr. F.M. -- Why Many Men Are Old at 40
SMITH, Parkinson E. -- Marriage, Sex and the Family
STIEGLITZ, Julius -- Chemistry in Medicine
SQUIBB, E.R. & Sons -- Squibb Product Reference For the Medical Profession
STONE, Chester T., M.D. -- The Dangerous Age in Men
SOCIETE DE CHIRURGIE DE LYON -- Lyon Chirurgical
SWARTOUT, Hubert O., M.D., Ph.D. -- Modern Medical Counselor
SWERN, Daniel -- Bailey's Industrial Oil and Fat Products (Third Edition)
TABER, Clarence Wilbur -- Taber's Cyclopedic Medical Dictionary
VON NOORDEN, Prof. Carl -- Disorders of Metabolism and Nutrition
WALLING, Prof. Wm. H., M.A., M.D. -- Sexology
WARMBRAND, Max, N.D., D.O. -- The Encyclopedia of Natural Health
WEST, Edward Staunton, Ph.D. and TODD, Wilbert R., Ph.D. -- Textbook of Biochemistry

Articles

ALLISON, Gene -- Health and Nutrition
BEREGOFF-GILLOW, Pauline, M.D. -- Urination -- "Herald of Health"
BRITISH MEDICAL JOURNAL -- Tuberculous Prostatitis and Vesiculitis

BRITISH MEDICAL JOURNAL --
Stilboestrol and Prostatic Enlargement
CHASE, Alice, D.O. -- Prostatism
CLEMENTS, S. Philip -- Prostate Troubles -- "Heal Thyself"
CUTOLO, S.R., M.D. -- Prostate Trouble Afflicts 50% of Men Over 50 -- "Rx Health"
DE KRUIF, Paul -- Prostate Trouble -- "The Reader's Digest"
THE EAGLE -- Homosexual Society Status Spurs Congressional Hearings
GRAY, Mary -- Prostate Gland Troubles -- "Health & You"
HAMILTON, Frank B., B. Sc., Ph.D. -- The Prostate - the "Male Womb" -- "Let's Live"
HART, James Pirie, B.Sc., and
COOPER, William Legrande, M.D. -- Vitamin F in the Treatment of Prostatic Hypertrophy
JONES, Wade Hampton -- Help for Prostate Trouble -- "Frontiers of Health"
LET'S LIVE -- Prostate gland enlargement
LIEF, Dr. Stanley -- Prostate Troubles - Their Causes and Treatment -- "Hamdard"
MOYLE, Alan, M.B.N.O.A. -- Self-Help For Prostate Sufferers -- "Health for All"
PORUDOMINSKY, Prof. E.M., M.D. -- Here's What the Doctor Says About Prostate Trouble -- "Northern Neighbors"
POWELL, Eric F. -- Prostate Enlargement -- "Fitness and the Gardener"
QUICK, Clifford, M.Sc., D.O., M.B.N.O.A. -- Prostate Troubles, How to Overcome Them -- "Health for All"

RAINES, Samuel L., M.D. -- Prostatic Cancer - More Cures with Earlier Detection -- "Consultant"
RICHES, E.W., M.S., F.R.C.S. -- Enlarged Prostate -- "British Medical Journal"
RODALE, J.I. -- Nutritional Therapy for Prostate Disorders -- "Prevention"
RODALE, J.I. -- The Prostate -- "Prevention"
RODALE, J.I. -- Is There a Male "Change of Life"? -- "Prevention"
RODALE, Robert -- Theory Links Heart Disease With Spices -- "Health Bulletin"
RODALE, Robert -- Arguments over Headache Drug Continue -- "Health Bulletin"
SAYEED, A.S. -- The Prostate Gland -- "Health and You"
SCHUTZER, A.I. -- Chilling Facts About the Gland That Makes You a Man -- "Mechanix Illustrated"
SCIENCE NEWS LETTER -- False 'Senility' Cured
SHELTON, Dr. Herbert M. -- Frequent Nocturnal Urination in Vegetarians -- "Hygienic Review"

Correspondence

Bartram, T.
Brenner, Joseph
Clements, George R.
Eley, William F., D. C.
Ellis, Wm. A., D.O.
Gehman, Dr. Jesse Mercer
Gillanders, H.E., B.A., M.D., C.M.

Gruner, O.C.
Hanoka, Dr. N.S.
Husted, H.H., O.D.
Jones, K.
Klein, Dr. Leo
Krok, Morris
Reeds, R. Robert, M.D.
Renner, John H., M.D.
Salmon, M.C.
Shelton, Herbert M., Ph.D.
Thomson, C. Leslie, B.Sc.
Warmbrand, Dr. Max
Wigmore, Ann, D.D.

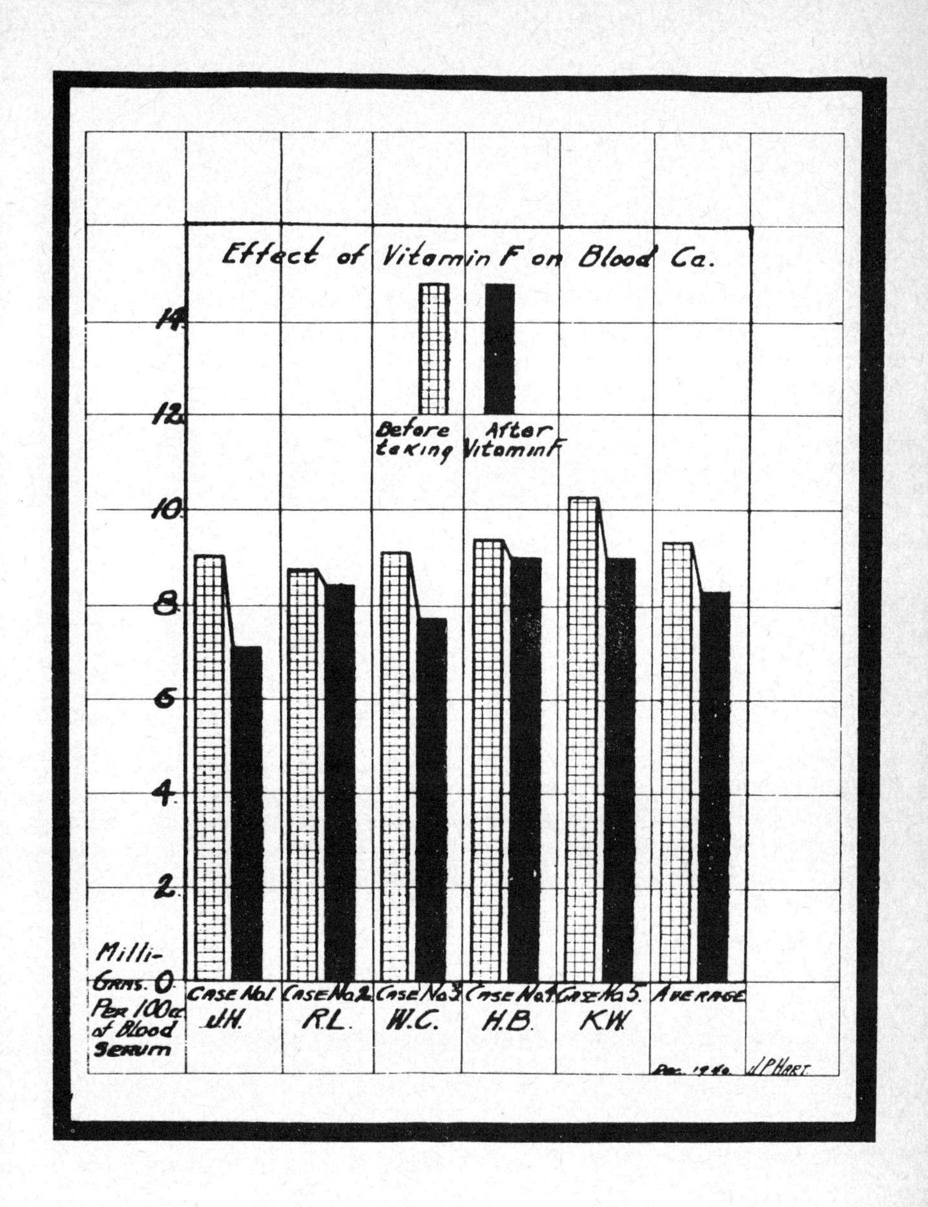

EFFECT OF VITAMIN F ON BLOOD CALCIUM